PRAISE FOR *THE ART OF HEALING*

"Behind the visible world of the body lies an invisible, unconscious domain that can be a powerful force in healing. Dr. Bernie Siegel is a pioneer in teaching individuals to bring this factor into conscious awareness. The result can be not only physical healing, but also peace, fulfillment, and joyful living. When we combine the art of healing with the science of curing, modern medicine becomes whole. Thanks, Bernie, for showing the way."

— Larry Dossey, MD, author of *One Mind*

"Bernie Siegel was already a very successful surgeon when he discovered the subtle forms of communication the human mind is capable of. He started to explore the unconscious, the work of Carl Jung, and the power to heal which is innate in all living things. He began a journey that resulted in more of his patients getting well. It caused him to change the direction of his career and to begin writing about what he had learned. With this latest book he tempers scientific knowledge with compassion as he uses his trained professional eye to take a warm and personal look at how perception, intention, and nonverbal/psychic communication affect healing and well-being.... This upbeat new book is full of ways in which [readers] can learn to better access and utilize that power for themselves."

— Anna Jedrziewski, *Retailing Insight*

PRAISE FOR *A BOOK OF MIRACLES*
BY BERNIE S. SIEGEL, MD

"As these stories show, love and magic can find us in any situation, no matter how difficult. This warm, uplifting book opens the door to seeing the miracles that are happening all around us, every day."

— Gerald Jampolsky, MD, author of *Love Is Letting Go of Fear*

"A call to take an evolutionary leap not through some kind of automatic unfoldment but by using conscious choice. Love, intelligence, and creativity are seeds waiting to be touched and awakened. The more you touch them, the more they flourish."

— Deepak Chopra, author of *The Seven Spiritual Laws of Success*

PRAISE FOR *365 PRESCRIPTIONS FOR THE SOUL*
BY BERNIE S. SIEGEL, MD

"Bernie Siegel dispenses spiritual medicine that's good for you, and feels good too! I highly recommend these daily doses of eternal wisdom."

— Marianne Williamson, author of *Everyday Grace*

"Bernie is one of the world's most respected doctors. I would pay close attention to any prescription he offers. I read from this each day."

— Wayne Dyer, author of *Getting in the Gap*

"Dr. Siegel's soul medicine is dispensed in perfect doses to uplift, inspire, enlighten, and heal you. As always, Bernie's wisdom and love gave me goosebumps, or should I say god-bumps. Buy a carton of this medicine-in-a-book and administer it to everyone you love."

— Joan Borysenko, PhD, author of *Inner Peace for Busy People*

PRAISE FOR *101 EXERCISES FOR THE SOUL*
BY BERNIE S. SIEGEL, MD

"Another loving, wise, practical, and life-changing book from Dr. Bernie. This step-by-step fitness guide is for the part of you that has wings."

— Rachel Naomi Remen, MD, author of *Kitchen Table Wisdom*

"This simple book has all the wisdom you need to live life from your best self. Bernie has the gift of taking complex ideas and making them simple and accessible. Follow his workout plan, and you'll create a life more wonderful than any you might ever have imagined."

— Joan Borysenko, PhD, author of *Inner Peace for Busy People*

"From one of America's master healers, a practical guide that provides a step-by-step entry into a healthier, more fulfilling way of being. Siegel is a genius for inspiring people to reach beyond themselves and attain what they thought not possible."

— Larry Dossey, MD, author of *Healing Words*

"A beautiful, heartfelt book by a legendary physician to help you nurture mind, body, and soul."

— Judith Orloff, MD, author of *Second Sight* and *Positive Energy*

"I have always admired Dr. Bernie Siegel as one of the most remarkable minds of our time. He combines an analytical scientific mind with a deep knowingness of spirituality. His *101 Exercises for the Soul* will help you understand and learn from that part of you which is the ultimate and supreme genius and mirrors the wisdom of the universe."

— Deepak Chopra, author of *The Book of Secrets*

"Dr. Siegel's inspiring exercises for achieving enlightenment in daily life bring together the wisdom of the ages into one crisp, precise, and highly readable book. It's a valuable addition to every spiritual traveler's essential library."

— Allen and Linda Anderson, authors of *Angel Dogs* and *Horses with a Mission*

THE ART OF HEALING

OTHER BOOKS BY BERNIE S. SIEGEL, MD

101 Exercises for the Soul
365 Prescriptions for the Soul
A Book of Miracles
Faith, Hope & Healing
Help Me to Heal
How to Live between Office Visits
Love, Magic & Mudpies
Love, Medicine & Miracles
Peace, Love & Healing
Prescriptions for Living

CHILDREN'S BOOKS
Buddy's Candle
Smudge Bunny

POETRY
Words & Swords

THE ART OF HEALING

UNCOVERING YOUR INNER WISDOM
AND POTENTIAL FOR SELF-HEALING

BERNIE S. SIEGEL, MD

WITH CYNTHIA J. HURN

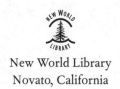

New World Library
Novato, California

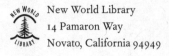

New World Library
14 Pamaron Way
Novato, California 94949

Text design by Tona Pearce Myers

Library of Congress Cataloging-in-Publication Data
Siegel, Bernie S.
 The art of healing : uncovering your inner wisdom and potential for self-healing /
Dr. Bernie S. Siegel with Cynthia J. Hurn.
    pages cm
Includes bibliographical references and index.
ISBN 978-1-60868-185-3 (pbk.) — ISBN 978-1-60868-186-0 (ebook)
 1. Mental healing. 2. Consciousness. 3. Spiritual healing. 4. Mind and body.
 5. Self-care, Health. I. Hurn, Cynthia. II. Title.
RZ400.S6215 2013
615.8'528—dc23   2013012986

First printing, September 2013
ISBN 978-1-60868-185-3
Printed in Canada on 100% postconsumer-waste recycled paper

New World Library is proud to be a Gold Certified Environmentally Responsible Publisher. Publisher certification awarded by Green Press Initiative. www.greenpressinitiative.org

10 9 8 7 6 5 4 3 2 1

Contents

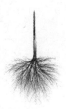

Acknowledgments

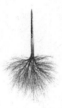

I thank and acknowledge the work of Cindy Hurn and Georgia Hughes, as well as the assistance of my agent, Andrea Hurst, in creating this book.

I also must acknowledge those who have been my life coaches and teachers: my wife, Bobbie; our children, Jonathan, Jeffrey, Stephen, Carolyn, and Keith, and their families; and all my four-legged friends, who are too numerous to list.

BERNIE SIEGEL, MD

Introduction

THE BIG QUESTIONS

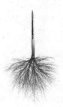

And therefore, if the head and body are to be well,
you must begin by curing the soul; that is the first thing.

— PLATO

Yesterday I went to get my driver's license renewed. I anticipated lines and the usual long wait with everybody wishing they could get out of there, so I wasn't looking forward to it. But soon after I arrived, a woman at the counter called my number. I looked around, surprised. Many of these people had waited much longer than I had; it had to be somebody else's turn. But she called out my number a second time, so I went up.

As soon as I got to the counter, a smile of recognition spread across her face. It turned out that I had operated on her mother many years ago. We had such a wonderful time talking and she shared how well her mother was doing. When I left she was still thanking me for helping her mother to heal. She wasn't referring to the surgery or the chemo-therapy. She was talking about her mother's *life*. Imagine that. It wasn't about her physical body or the disease; it was about the things that made her mother's life meaningful. When I left there, I felt so good. Our meeting had not been an accident or by chance. It was a gift. There are no coincidences.

What I am about to share — what led me to a new understanding of the nature of life — stems not from my beliefs but from my personal experience and my work with patients and their families. My attitude of keeping an open mind allowed me to gain much more from my experi-ences and become a better healer than those in the profession who say they can't accept what they can't understand or explain. If we don't seek knowledge, we don't learn; we lose the opportunity to live our lives in a creative way. So I never stopped asking the important ques-tions. What do I mean by the important questions?

The questions we must ask are: How does the invisible become vis-ible? What part of our being still sees when we leave our physical body in a near-death experience? How do we intuitively know what plans our unconscious mind is creating? How do clairvoyants and psychics communicate with people and animals, whether distant or dead? How does the community of cells in the body speak to the conscious mind about its needs and health? And what is the language of creation and the soul?

The invisible I talk about is what lies within our physical, mental, emotional, and psychic body. Most of us become aware of our inner harmony or disharmony through moods, feelings, and symptoms, and we rely on medical examinations and lab tests to know what is hap-pening inside the body. But imagine if we were able to know *before* a physical affliction or emotional breakdown awakened us. How much healthier we would be and how much fuller our lives would become. Because of physicians' limited medical training, rarely do we have the option to learn about the true cause of disease. And yet it is possible to prevent disease and emotional breakdown.

If we take the lid off our unconscious, we can be guided by a deeper knowing. The practices and techniques of going within allow us to communicate with and learn from the greater intelligence, whether we choose to do so through spontaneous drawings, dreams, meditation, breath work, or any number of practices that place us within the healing realm of our inner wisdom.

Communication with the greater intelligence is not only possible, but it also happens all the time whether we are aware of it, and tuned into it, or not. The same intelligence that allows cells to communicate inside the human body is inherent in all life-forms. It is characterized by its fluidity and moves with both intention and abandon, crossing all barriers of matter, time, and space. It serves us in ways that often seem like coincidence. Unexplained happenings, healings, and lifesaving or comforting messages appear just at the moment you need them, as happened to me yesterday, when my wait to renew my driver's license was cut short and ended with the gift of gratitude.

To be receptive to this communication, whether it comes to you through symbols or words, you must quiet your mind, like a still pond, with no turbulence to obscure its reflections. Today was a good example. I'm the caregiver for my wife, Bobbie, who has been living with multiple sclerosis for several decades. There are days when I have my hands so full of caregiving and other responsibilities that everything seems overwhelming. It's a challenge sometimes to love my fate and learn the lesson of compassion. While devoting most of my life to healing people, I have encouraged them to care for themselves as well as they do for others. But living the sermon can be hard to do when you're providing long-term care for someone you love. It's easy to forget that you too have needs.

This morning, I took the dogs for a walk in one of my favorite places. The cemetery near our house is several centuries old. It's out in the suburbs, and rarely do I meet anybody there, unless it's the anniversary of somebody's death or a funeral is taking place. Because the cemetery is so peaceful, I can let the dogs run around. For me, it's like a walking meditation, and for them it's an adventure. Dogs are masters of living in the moment. Today the dogs discovered something on the ground, not close to a grave but lying beside the road. I went over and picked it up. It was a tiny white teddy bear with the message *Love Me* on its chest. The bear was as clean and unmarked as if it had just come off the store shelf. I looked around the cemetery; there wasn't a person in sight. I read the words again out loud: *Love Me*. I felt as if somebody had put it there knowing that this was the message I needed. It was such a gift. I put the bear in my pocket and took it home.

Apparent coincidences like this one happen exactly when they are most needed. When you allow yourself quiet moments, you increase the opportunity to receive messages of love and support. The little bear now sits on the kitchen counter with other teddy bears I have found. I create shrines with them in our home to give me therapy all day long.

The language of creation and the soul is expressed in many ways, sometimes in a subtle whisper, other times spoken so clearly, it is difficult to doubt, let alone ignore. I used to be a skeptic because I didn't know any better. I wasn't trained to look through any other lens. But over time, I learned to open my mind to other kinds of communication and possibilities. I have had an animal intuitive locate our lost cat in Connecticut while she sat in California. I have had a near-death experience and, through this, learned that we are more than our bodies. I have had past-life experiences and had messages from dead patients delivered to me through mediums. I have even heard the voices of the dead speak to me. I did not seek any of these experiences, but I have lived them. Rather than deny the reality of these occurrences on the basis that I could not understand them, I sought, like astronomers and physicists, to accept what I experienced, explore the invisible, and communicate with it.

The psychotherapist Ernest Rossi has observed that "our daily and hourly life experiences, sensations, thoughts, images, emotions and behavior can modulate gene expression and neurogenesis in ways that actually can change the physical structure and functioning of our brain."[1] What he meant is that your mind is like a remote control with an infinite number of channels to choose from (the greater consciousness), and your body is like the TV screen that plays whichever channels you tune in to. If you limit yourself to the channels accepted by your peers, your life will be all about staying within the boundaries of their discipline, and your measure of success will be based on the amount of recognition you have achieved. In other words, if you pay attention to the money channel rather than the spiritual channel, your life becomes all about material things, and your measure of success is based on what you have accumulated. If you pay attention to the spiritual channel, your life then focuses on improving the world, and your measure of success is based on what you have done to enhance life. You are no longer governed by social, political, and religious rules and regulations. Your life, which was God's gift to you, becomes your gift to God through your actions.

Consciousness can be experienced as a universal field that affects us all, and studies by quantum physicists have verified this. Books such as *The Psychobiology of Gene Expression*, by Rossi, give insight to the process by which the universal mind works. Rossi refers to a form of intelligence that communicates through changes in our genes. He writes, "This special class of genes [immediate early genes] can respond to psychosocial cues and significant life events in an adaptive manner within minutes. Immediate early genes have been described as the newly discovered mediators between nature and nurture: they receive signals from the environment to activate genes that code for the formation of proteins, which then carry out the adaptive functions of the cell in health and illness. Immediate early genes integrate mind and body; they are key players in psychosomatic medicine, mind-body healing, and the therapeutic arts."[2]

If you have trouble believing that genes can act to communicate important messages that initiate immediate survival responses, think about how bacteria learn to resist antibiotics, viruses resist antivirals, the wounds of living things heal, living things resist parasites, and more. All of these processes require a form of intelligence that grasps the situation and then communicates a desired response to the rest of the body's cells. And this needs to be done at the level of genes if the knowledge is to be passed to future generations.

Knowledge and memories are stored not only in our brains but also in the cells of our bodies. This becomes most apparent when a recipient of an organ transplant awakens from surgery with new, unique memories and some preferences of the person whose organ is now within her body. Soon after Claire Sylvia had her heart-lung transplant operation at Yale–New Haven Hospital, she was asked what she wanted more than anything else, and she said, "Actually, I'm dying for a beer right now."[3] She asked herself, why did I say that? She never drank beer; she didn't even *like* beer. It so happened that the donated heart had come from a beer-loving teenager who rode motorcycles. Later he came to her in a dream and told her his name. Eventually she found the family through their son's obituary, got to know them, and learned more about their son. Claire, whom I discuss further in chapter 4, asked me to come and see her because, although everybody thought she was crazy, she knew I would listen to her. She wrote a book about her experience, *A Change of Heart*.

Another form of invisible intelligence and communication outside the body is discussed in Lynne McTaggart's book *The Field*. She writes, "Quantum physicists had discovered a strange property in the subatomic world called 'nonlocality.' This [property is] the ability of a quantum entity such as an individual electron to influence another quantum particle instantaneously over any distance *despite there being no exchange of force or energy*." Once any form of contact happens between quantum particles, they "retain a connection even when separated, so that the actions of one will always influence the other, no matter how far they get separated."[4]

Evidence of invisible communication between particles smaller than atoms has been around for a long time. For example, biological mutations that happen within one variety of plant in one part of the world have also been recorded happening in the same variety of plant in other parts of the world. Knowledge is communicated, too, such as when a species of animal learns to use a stick as a tool for a specific task and the skill is learned at the same time in other parts of the world, within the species, even though no visible means of communication or physical connection has taken place.

In England, after many years of milk delivery, birds suddenly learned to peck open milk containers that had been delivered to people's homes. During World War II, milk deliveries were cancelled. When the war ended and milk was again left on people's doorsteps, the birds immediately began to peck open the containers. Due to the length of time involved, few of the latter group of birds had been alive when the milk deliveries ceased. How could the untrained youngsters so quickly understand what to do?

Once physicists identified nonlocality (the subatomic property of quantum particles influencing other particles without using physical exchange of force or energy), observers recognized that it explained certain phenomena, such as animals knowing skills they were never taught. What traveled across the world and across generations was not matter but intelligence.

In Western medicine, when doctors hear about something that wasn't a part of their education or training, they often say, "I can't accept that." What they mean is: "I can't explain it." So they reject it. But if we want to utilize our potential, we need to keep an open mind. William Bengston, PhD, in his book, *The Energy Cure: Unraveling the Mystery of Hands-On Healing*, wrote about his experimental research on mice that had been injected with an aggressive cancer with a 100 percent track record of becoming terminal in a matter of weeks. Bengston trained student researchers to perform a hands-on healing technique called image cycling. The researchers had never practiced healing, nor did they have any interest or faith in it. In the majority of cases, the mice were completely healed of the disease. This result happened not once but many times over during the controlled experiments in the science laboratories of several highly respected institutions. Even Bengston's peers who had observed the experiments, seen the controls, and witnessed the amazing results refused to believe that traditional medicine would ever take his work seriously.[5]

Near-death experiences tell us we are more than just physical bodies. Jung often said that psyche and matter are complementary aspects of the same thing. I believe these two aspects communicate with each other through images, the language of creation and intention. We can, through the images in our dreams and spontaneous drawings, tap our inner wisdom and reveal the authentic person we are truly meant to be. We can remove negative messages that have been implanted in our minds and retrain our thoughts using creative visualization and positive affirmations to adopt life-promoting attitudes. We can learn how to live in the moment and utilize the healing power of daily practices such as laughter, meditation, and journaling. Loving and healing our lives is not only about dismantling disease: it is also about being healthy, at peace, and fulfilled.

In *The Art of Healing*, I discuss all of these topics as well as the benefits that can be gained from working with, and learning from, animals, psychics, and intuitives. While sharing actual patients' stories, I hope to illustrate on a practical level how others have incorporated creative practices with positive results. Throughout the book, I also offer a variety of prescriptive exercises (each labeled "Doctor's Rx") to help you explore your own inner world of wisdom.

Since giving up surgery to help my patients heal in a different way, I have referred to myself as a "Jungian surgeon." I now use tools other than surgical instruments to help patients. A box of crayons, a water gun, a noisemaker, and a Magic Marker became four of those tools. You will read about the formation of the Exceptional Cancer Patients therapy group that my wife, Bobbie, and I started. The group still meets regularly and has helped hundreds of patients heal their lives as well as their bodies. People have the potential built into them to induce self-healing. Time and again I have seen my patients experience many positive results when they adopted some of the techniques and attitudes covered in this book.

On my website, berniesiegelmd.com, I offer books and meditation CDs, as well as individual guidance in the section "Ask Bernie a Question." In the many articles and interviews posted on the site, I recommend creative tools that guide people in the decision-making process they use in their day-to-day lives and when confronting a variety of challenges. This book, *The Art of Healing*, is meant to augment these tools, helping people learn how to live (or die) in harmony, wholeness, and peace.

I want to share my method of Jungian surgery with the world, particularly with health care professionals and with patients and their families so they will come to understand how somatic aspects of health and disease are inseparable from the natural integration of mind, body, and spirit. We spend a lot of time and money exploring outer space, but inner space offers the same wonder and mystery, and it should be included in our medical professionals' education.

When we open our minds, when we listen to and draw from our inner wisdom and the greater consciousness, we begin the fulfilling and sometimes miraculous journey toward health and self-induced healing. When we agree to take this journey, we become the artists, and our lives, the canvas. I invite you now to adopt the curiosity and openness of a child. Take my hand and walk with me through these pages. You will soon discover as we work together that you have been creating, practicing, and experiencing the art of healing. When the artist is alive within us, we become stimulating, creative beings from whom everyone around us can benefit. So read on, pick up your brush and palette, and start living your authentic life.

Chapter 1

THE DOCTOR'S AWAKENING

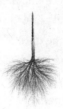

*Buried within the subconscious, in the farthest corner of our memory,
lies the knowledge of everything we need to know about living.*

— RABBI NOAH WEINBERG

*I*magine what it is like to look into the eyes of a person as you tell him, "You've got Stage IV cancer." His whole life is now turned upside down. You see the expression in his eyes and in the eyes of the loved ones who have accompanied him. Imagine what it is like when your patient is alone, with no one there to support her when she gets the news. In either case, you are that patient's lifeline and their source of hope. You are their life coach on the road to survival and can help them achieve their potential through self-induced healing.

I became a physician because I like people and I wanted to help them get well when they were ill. But after years of practicing as a pediatric and general surgeon and performing many operations, I felt overwhelmed with the realization that I could not fix or cure all of my patients. I was in a lot of pain with nobody to talk to about it. I was also angry that my education as a doctor had not prepared me to deal with people's lives; it had only taught me about the mechanics of medicine and surgery. I even wrote to the deans of the medical school I attended, saying: you made me a wonderful technician, but you did not teach me how to take care of myself or my patients.

A retired physician who went to divinity school and became a chaplain at the Yale School of Medicine did a study in which he asked surgeons, as part of his research, how it felt to be a surgeon. With each respondent, he had to repeat the question three to five times before he or she stopped saying, "*I think....*" When these surgeons finally used the words *I feel*, most of them said it felt painful and admitted they did not want to get to know their patients.

Many other studies have revealed that surgeons have a higher rate of depression, burnout, and suicidal ideation than the general population, and that when a surgical error is made, or surgery is not successful in curing the patient, surgeons suffer even more. They are also the least likely of those in high-stress professions (such as police, social workers, teachers, and nurses) to seek counseling or psychological help.

Trying to avoid emotional pain, surgeons often distance themselves from their patients and refer to them by their diagnosis or disease, hospital room number, or treatment. I've heard doctors discuss patients with their colleagues and refer to them as "the double mastectomy" or "the glioblastoma," even when standing within earshot of the patient. What picture comes to mind when I say "the double mastectomy?" Do you see the face of a woman who has a family, a husband, and children who love her? No. You see only her deformity and the scarring of her body.

I believe a doctor who sees patients without knowing how to listen to and communicate with them is like a minister who doesn't know how to talk with God. When a patient feels that his surgeon doesn't see him as a human being, both the disease and its treatment become sources of greater fear; feelings of isolation and powerlessness can settle in a patient's mind and affect his ability to survive.

The longer I practiced as a surgeon, the harder it became for me not to feel as if I'd failed my patients and myself. I couldn't understand why God made such an imperfect world. In 1977, I heard about a workshop called "Psychological Factors, Stress and Cancer," which was presented by Carl Simonton, a radiation oncologist.

During the early years of Dr. Simonton's career, he observed that when patients with similar cancers were given the same dose of radiation, the outcomes of their radiation treatments varied considerably. He identified the variables between the patients and found that the only statistically significant difference appeared to be in the patients' attitudes and will to live. He concluded that people with a more positive attitude generally lived longer and suffered fewer side effects from the radiation.

Simonton added lifestyle counseling, which included meditation and mental imagery, to his therapeutic techniques, and he helped to break through the rigid mold of established medical practices at that time. The results of his research indicated that when lifestyle counseling was incorporated into the medical treatment plan for patients with advanced cancer, their survival time doubled and their quality of life improved. Simonton published the results of his studies in medical journals and in *Getting Well Again*, a book he coauthored with his wife, Stephanie Matthews-Simonton (a psychologist), and James Creighton.[1]

I was excited to attend Simonton's seminar and looked forward to learning skills that would help me and my patients. I had presumed the event was designed for physicians and other people in the medical field, and I was shocked to discover that I was the only physician in the room. With the exception of two psychologists, all the other attendees were cancer patients.

In my work as a surgeon, I would often visualize a surgical procedure in great detail the day before the operation, preparing myself for the anatomical structures I would be working around and predicting what challenges might arise during surgery, but I had no previous experience of guided mental imagery. I was somewhat skeptical, then, when Carl Simonton played soft music and told his listeners to close their eyes. I was seated next to one of my patients in the front of the room, and when Carl looked at me I didn't want him to think I wasn't complying, so I closed my eyes. When Carl said, "You will see your inner guide approaching you...," I thought, "This is nuts; I didn't come here for this."

I'm an artist — a painter — which means I'm a visual person. Despite my initial skepticism, I closed my eyes and followed Carl's voice, and soon I began to walk through the guided imagery, visualizing with clarity and great detail. The experience I had was incredible. Suddenly it was no longer a matter of: What do I believe? Instead it was: What did I experience?

During each of the exercises we participated in, my mind opened to things I had not been exposed to in my professional training; the lens of my perception began to change. I watched in fascination as workshop participants visibly relaxed and expressions of happiness, hope, and serenity transformed their faces. Rather than feel like victims of their disease, patients came to realize they had powerful inner resources for healing and problem solving.

In 1979, I returned to my office after only three days at another seminar, one run by Elisabeth Kübler-Ross. By the end of the day, one of my partners, Dr. Richard Selzer, said to me, "You're gone."

I asked, "What do you mean?"

"You're a totally different person," he said. "You are going to leave surgery."

He could sense the change in my consciousness and intuitively saw what I couldn't. He was right. Within ten years I retired from surgery to talk to people and help heal in another way. How did he know what was in my future? What intuition spoke to him, and where did it come from?

When I attended the Kübler-Ross seminar, the work we did with spontaneous drawings revealed, in a matter of hours, incredible insights and information about my life. Because of my training as a surgeon and my knowledge of anatomy, I was also seeing things in the drawings people made that a psychotherapist would not normally be aware of, particularly the structure of various disease states and of treatments that were unconsciously being revealed in those drawings. Subconscious leaks of information appeared in normal objects like trees, clouds, and people, and they showed the patient's authentic physical, emotional, and spiritual state; the images became symbols of each person's inner and outer truth. While there I learned that Carl Jung was fascinated by individuals' subconscious knowledge about the body and the psyche as revealed in his patients' drawings.

It was then that I became a believer, and a box of crayons became one of my therapeutic tools. I began to ask my patients and their families to draw pictures. These would help us to make therapeutic decisions based not simply on intellect but on inner knowingness, and would help us understand family relationships and psychological issues. I soon became angry that the significance of drawings and dreams, as they relate to physical and psychological factors, is not routinely taught in medical school. I have yet to meet a medical student or physician who was told during training that Carl Jung was able to diagnose a brain tumor from a patient's dream.[2]

When I realized how much knowledge I lacked, despite the number of years I had spent in medical school, I made contact with Jungian therapists to explore their work and wisdom. Gregg Furth, a Jungian psychologist and the author of *The Secret World of Drawings*,[3] helped to guide me, as did another Jungian psychologist, Susan Bach, author of *Life Paints Its Own Span*. She based her book on her studies of drawings made by children with leukemia. She too had become aware that both psychological and physical aspects were revealed in the children's drawings. The somatic or organic clues aided in reaching their diagnosis, treating the child, and developing a prognosis, and they became an important means of communication for the doctor, patient, and family.[4]

I will never forget a note I received from Bach after I wrote to tell her what I had discovered in my patients' drawings. She wrote back: "Calm down; we know all this." Psychologists had long been seeing a change in people's physical health when they got their lives in order. In my excitement, I also wrote to editors of American psychological journals, and was told that this information was "appropriate but not interesting," while the editors of medical journals told me it was "interesting but not appropriate" for their publications. The reaction of the former editors, along with Susan Bach's response, confirmed to me that there was consistency in what was known and accepted by mental health professionals across the world.

Before attending the workshops, when I thought about my patients I would see their cancers. I would focus on the physical aspects of their diseases and take on the burden of responsibility to fix them. After the workshops, I began to visualize my patients as human beings who have the capacity and potential to heal. I took more time to listen to them and asked more questions, such as "Can you describe for me what you are feeling and experiencing?" Words like *confusion*, *failure*, and *draining* would pour out of them. If my patient said, "It's like pressure on my back and shoulders," I would ask him, "What is happening in your life that could be described as pressure and is creating pressure for you?" Inevitably the patient would talk about a current or recent circumstance in his life that he associated with the feeling of carrying a burden or being trapped by the weight of responsibility. The mental connection between his emotion and his physical state made it possible for him to explore ways of making changes that would ease his burden and give his body a better chance to heal. Some patients began to heal when they saw their disease as a blessing, a wake-up call, or new beginning.

A DIFFERENT APPROACH

Now that I was focusing on the positive aspects of my patients and the goals we aimed to achieve, I no longer felt isolated and burdened with responsibility. One of my patients had said to me at the Simonton workshop, "Bernie, I feel better when I'm in the office with you, but I can't take you home with me. I need to know how to live between office visits." When she said that, I thought, Wow, I don't have to feel like a failure. Even if I can't cure their diseases, but can help people to live, I've done something for them. So I sent out letters to a hundred of our patients with cancer, saying, "If you want to live and have a longer, better life, come to a meeting."

I had no idea how many people would respond to the letter. At the time, I was thinking, "If I had cancer and my doctor sent me a letter asking if I wanted to try something new, wouldn't I tell everyone I knew with cancer to come to the meeting?"

A few hours before the event was scheduled to begin, I panicked. I was imagining several hundred people showing up and forming a long line outside the building. How would I seat them all? My wife, Bobbie, who was helping to facilitate the workshop, reminded me that all ventures must begin somewhere, somehow, and no matter what happened, at least we were moving in a positive direction. She cracked a few of her one-liners, and our laughter helped me to relax.

By the appointed time, fewer than a dozen women had shown up. I couldn't believe it. I realized I would have to accept that I just didn't know the degree of my patients' will to live or their real motivations and desires. My wife said that since the majority of my cancer patients received the invitation but ignored the opportunity for something free that might help them, the people who did attend must be exceptional patients, and so she named the new group Exceptional Cancer Patients (ECaP).

My patients became my teachers. One of the most important things they taught me is that exceptional behavior is something we are all capable of, and that when we learn how to practice it we become aware of our own healing potential. Members of ECaP have experienced so many physical, spiritual, and psychological benefits, that many of them earned a reputation among my hospital colleagues as being "one of Bernie's crazy patients." Doctors were overheard saying, "That group of Bernie's — they seem a little nuts, but they keep getting well," and so the description "one of Bernie's crazy patients" became a compliment.

ECaP continues today. It is a synthesis of individual and group therapy that utilizes meditation, creative visualization, spontaneous drawings, dreams, humor, and the exploration of feelings. It is based on *carefrontation*: a safe, loving, and therapeutic confrontation, which facilitates personal lifestyle changes, personal empowerment, and healing of the individual's life.

More than thirty years after ECaP began, cancer centers across the country are, I'm happy to say, utilizing some form of multimethod therapeutic group work. The need for encouraging more of a mind-body-spirit approach in traditional medicine is still great, especially in the training of medical professionals. But scientific research and attitudes are slowly changing, and the direction of change has often been positive.

In this book, I hope to offer not only information but also inspiration. In each chapter, I give theoretical background backed up by stories of patients, and I suggest exercises that offer you a chance to experience each of these complementary healing tools.

Chapter 2

SOURCE, SIGNIFICANCE, AND VALIDITY OF SYMBOLS

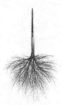

*When the soul wants to experience something,
she throws out an image in front of her and then steps into it.*

— MEISTER ECKHART

I often marvel at the intelligence within seeds, wondering what image of life they hold in their cells. How does a seed know what it is to become and how to nourish its growth? What impresses me even more is seeing a sprout pushing up through pavement. How do seeds know which way is up when light and warmth are blocked? And why don't they give up when they realize they have been paved over and are hitting a stone wall? I have used examples of plant behavior to inspire my family and patients. Plants possess a source of wisdom in their genes and a sense of gravity too. They don't give in to adversity when they run into obstacles; they push forward or find new ways to reach the light. So what signals plants to keep going and not succumb to obstacles?

The key to all forms of life is *communication*. This includes the ability of simple, one-celled organisms as well as the more complex ones, such as humans, to communicate with each other. It also refers to the exchange of information between systems, organs, and cells within individual bodies, and with the greater consciousness that is behind all creation.

Cellular communication evolved when one-celled organisms discovered how to pass on vital information by altering the chemistry of their environment. In times of danger they would secrete substances that led them to come together into balls of cells that could survive adverse living conditions such as droughts or temperature fluctuations. This clustering can also be seen in far more complex creatures, such as herd animals like elephants and even gray whales when they circle around and protect vulnerable members of the community from predatory attack.

Evolving organisms learned the difference between life-sustaining and self-destructive behavior at both conscious and unconscious levels, providing a pathway for the intelligence of their predecessors to be passed down to living individuals in each species. Problems arise for the human species when we do not pay attention to messages of danger because our *level of consciousness* distracts us. Notice I didn't say our intelligence.

If we grow up with life-enhancing, loving messages from the authorities in our lives, we respond to danger and preserve our health and lives because we have self-esteem. We behave with intelligence and pay attention to the unconscious signals we give our bodies and that they give us. But if we grow up with rejection, our choices and reactions become self-destructive, not life enhancing. When we respond appropriately to our bodies' signals, the intracellular communication becomes life enhancing; but when we ignore or deny the signals or we live in fear, they can be disease inducing.

Consider the man who continually says yes to overtime demands by his boss, ignoring the signals that say his body is wearing down from the stress of too much work. Disease may become his body's response when the man ignores signs of fatigue and abandons self-care, because the disease allows him to stop working. He may suffer from the Monday morning syndrome — named after the day in the week when people have more heart attacks, suicides, strokes, and illnesses. On the other hand, if he wakes up dreading the day and feels his blood pressure rise, and he listens to his body, he will realize that he must seek another, less stressful job — must find a job that he loves doing — or change his attitude toward his job and boss. When he changes the internal messages, his body will respond with renewed health.

One mechanism of communication is imagery. Before any information can be passed on, it must be organized into a pattern or code. This pattern may delineate a figure, as a sewing pattern does; the code may formulate a thought, much like the honey bee dancing to show her peers where nectar is, or it might predicate an action, such as when a traffic light turns green. Once an intention exists, an image is born and communication begins. Communication can be a simple message, such as when a cellular switch says, "Turn on" or "Turn off," or the message can be an intricate series of images that lead to the building of a cathedral, such as the one illustrated by my friend's story.

There is a stone cottage that sits at the edge of an ancient copse outside the cathedral city of Wells in England. When Harry bought the property, he discovered behind it the remains of an abandoned quarry, which had been the source of stone used to build Wells Cathedral in AD 1175. I was fascinated to learn from Harry that one part of his house had been the original quarryman's cottage, making the dwelling nearly a thousand years old.

"Beneath the tree roots and moss," he said, "I found giant slabs of stone with chisel marks still visible. Days later, when I stood under the magnificent arches of the cathedral, it struck me how incredible it was. Because of one man's imagination, desire, and intention, massive stones had been gouged from the earth, dragged five miles down the hill, and carved into pillars, walls, and the intricate, vaulted roof of the nave. I felt I was in the presence of the hand of God, seeing this miracle of creation manifested from one person's initial vision. Without man's ability to visualize and communicate complex ideas, no cathedral could or would have existed."

All species react to images at some level. What makes our species unique is not our ability to reason; it is the way we use images. Even those born without sight can respond to and interpret images and symbols. Reading Braille, for example, requires the ability to perceive and recognize specific shapes and patterns that contain a meaning.

When we evolved into humans, we became more complex in our interactions with the outer world. We developed language and created works of art. But still, in a wordless greater consciousness, we sought information from a universal intelligence that could only be conceived by visual, auditory, and tactile images, and we expressed what we learned with stories and symbols. Prehistoric drawings on cave walls and desert rocks, for example, illustrate visions that were sought by humans from an invisible source during times of drought. In other locations, shamans' illustrations provided passersby with information about how far and in what direction hunters would find life-supporting prey.

Symbols are a form of language that is understood without words and that acts as a mental shortcut. They may represent an object, a situation, a belief, a group of people, or many other possibilities. A symbol, such as the red octagonal traffic sign, may express only one meaning or, like a myth or parable, may be multilayered and deep. Such myths and parables are the symbolic stories that teach and that form the structure and beliefs of cultures and religions. These stories become embedded not only in the culture but also in the psyches of people.

Colors often share universal symbolism. People react to red with emotion (as they do to blood), to yellow as wake-up energy (sun), and to green as a positive indicator (growth). Not only does the symbolic meaning of the color affect what action we take, but it also communicates with our body, mind, and emotions at a subconscious level.

Gregg Furth writes in *The Secret World of Drawings*, "The symbol unlocks unconscious psychic energy and allows it to flow toward a natural level, where a transforming effect occurs. The individual encountering a difficulty now has the possibility of pulling unconscious elements into consciousness, dealing with them, and thus transcending the problem. The external problem may still be present, but it is now understood differently."[1] The new understanding is the key to growth and survival.

When words, sounds, and images become metaphors, they carry a greater meaning in a simple representation, such as the ring of a bell, and are capable of activating healing at the level of heart and mind. These symbols communicate with the body through feelings, mood, and automatic physical reactions. Symbolic images and their associated feelings can change our internal chemistry.

Followers of Buddhism, for example, learn to become aware of the stillness within at the sound of a ringing bell, their call to prayer and meditation. I often teach people to use the bell of a ringing phone as an opportunity for practicing mindfulness. One troubled woman who had adopted this practice was saved by the auditory prompt. Lost in the darkness of depression, she was just about to commit suicide when her telephone rang. The sound reminded her to go within and find that place of stillness. Once there, she realized she did not need to kill herself. She needed to learn how to live.

In the 1960s, Carl Jung's analytic approach to psychology transformed the understanding and attitudes of psychologists and sociologists in Europe and the United States. He studied the psyche through the worlds of dreams, art, mythology, religion, and philosophy. Although he was a practicing clinical psychologist, much of his life's work was spent exploring other realms, including Eastern and Western philosophy, alchemy, astrology, and sociology, as well as literature and the arts. His theory of the collective unconscious as expressed through symbols and archetypal characters opened the door to what is now referred to as Jungian psychology.

By Jung's definition, an archetype is a collectively understood, symbolic character shared among entire groups of people across epochs of time. These archetypal characters are the symbols of authority and key figures in our lives. The symbols alone have great influence on our feelings, thoughts, and behavior.[2]

Jung acknowledged that our future is shaped unconsciously. He also observed that we act as if we were gods controlling our lives, and that once we uncover the hidden realms inside us we discover that we are influenced and changed by many unseen factors. For further reading on this subject, I recommend Joseph Campbell's book *The Hero's Journey* and his documentary dialogue *The Power of Myth*.[3]

The Book of Changes, also called the I Ching, contains the wisdom of ancient Chinese sages who organized their observations of nature into sixty visual scenarios or objects. By tossing sticks or throwing coins, one creates a pattern made up of six broken or solid lines, and the resultant symbol, called a hexagram, represents one of the sixty images. The sages' written judgment and commentary on that hexagram is then used by the inquirer to gain insight into a problem or situation. I am amazed at what I have learned from it in times of need. In a recent time of change, it reminded me of my limitations and to act accordingly, helping me to remember that I cannot fix everything, and that I too have needs.

When Carl Jung was asked to write the foreword to the third edition of the English translation of the I Ching, he hesitated. He knew that, by introducing a system of divination in which one sought judgment from an ancient book upon a modern-day problem by tossing coins or casting sticks, he would incur criticism from his peers.

Having considered the risk to his respected reputation, Jung wrote, "I have always tried to remain unbiased and curious. Why not venture a dialogue with an ancient book that purports to be animated?" He decided to throw the coins and ask the book for its commentary on his "intention to present it to the western mind." The coin-tossing ritual produced a hexagon named the Cauldron, which represented "a ritual vessel containing cooked food. Here, the food is to be understood as spiritual nourishment."[4]

Many symbols in the I Ching would not have pertained to Jung's question; indeed, most would have been totally unrelated and the commentary deemed nonsense. But the sages' further discourse on the Cauldron was so applicable to Jung's query that he was encouraged to go ahead. He wrote the foreword, using his own experience with the coins as a reliable example of tapping into universal wisdom using an ancient Chinese method of symbols.

John Greenleaf Whittier, an active abolitionist and one of the American fireside poets, wrote, "Nature speaks in symbols and signs."[5] How often have you pondered a question and found your answer when gazing on feeding birds in the wild or watching a sunset? More than just metaphor or story, symbols can produce emotional reactions, induce healing, and act as transformative lessons.

One woman I knew battled with depression after she moved to the West Coast. Despite the beauty that surrounded her, she struggled against suicidal thoughts as she walked along the beach on a desolate reach of sand.

I had yearned to live in this place for so many years, but now that I was here, I felt terribly alone. I could see for miles, and there wasn't another human being in sight. I felt so depressed that if anyone had appeared I would have avoided them. That sense of isolation nearly overwhelmed me. I tried hard not to panic, and I kept saying "thank you" out loud, hoping gratitude would change my dark thoughts.

Just then a stone in the sand caught my eye. Smooth and flat, the stone was shaped like a perfectly cast footprint. I picked it up. Despite the cool weather and thick overcast sky, the stone contained the heat of the sun, and its warmth began to envelop me. I knew the footprint was a message meant especially for me, and I no longer felt alone. I also realized my sense of isolation had been brought on by my own choices.

Within the week I got involved with my community through volunteer work, and I started attending twelve-step meetings and making friends with other women in the program. There are still moments when I feel lonely, but when they happen I reach out to help someone else and walk beside another human being. The stone footprint sits on my desk as I write, reminding me of just how loved and un-alone I am.

For this woman, the stone represented a story about footprints in the sand; a story that has become a metaphor for God's presence. The symbol transformed her thinking; it offered comfort and a reminder that she had to take steps that would make her life meaningful.

I look for signs, too, and when I find a penny, I always feel I am on the right path. Engraved on each penny are the words "In God We Trust," which is a reminder for me to have faith, and the word "Liberty," a reminder to be my authentic self. Abe Lincoln reminds me of my mortality and also to lighten up a bit.

We know that cellular communication happens through chemical and electrical signals that direct the cell's behavior, but how a protein molecule knows what to do is beyond me. Creation is a miracle and is beyond our understanding. It is amazing to think of one cell — an ovum — developing into a human being, differentiating into all the components we are made of, getting them to know their role and to develop in the right place in the body to do their thing. Imagine the endless number of intercellular signals that have to be sent to each component of the body in the process of making a viable human being — a baby. And consider the signals this body receives after it is formed and throughout its lifespan.

What does a touch, a hug, or a caress say to that body about living? What do unexpressed feelings of fear, despair, and depression tell it about the desire to live? Every cell in our body is aware of our will to live and of our desires and intentions. The emotional and physical are one. Mind and matter are not separate entities. As Jung said, the psyche and soma are simply different aspects of the One Being we are.

Just as one-celled organisms react to their environments, our body cells react to physical, mental, and emotional environments both inside and outside the body. A negatively perceived image can be the path that directs us away from our intended journey; but when we turn it around and perceive it as positive, we can recover what ground we've lost and continue, strengthened and wiser, on life's journey.

Human beings perceive life from a dualistic perspective, through which we understand that where there is light, there is also shadow. However, a shadow is merely the absence of light. If you face the sun, you don't experience the shadow. Perception, then, affects our health; and most often, the way we perceive is our choice. Disease is a loss of health, not a punishment. Lost health is to be looked for and recovered, just as you would seek to find your lost car keys rather than assume God wanted you to walk home.

SYMBOLS OF HEALING

Consider the ancient symbol in which a serpent is entwined around a staff. Originally it signified Asclepius, the Greek god of healing and medicine. The rod, or staff, of Asclepius, adopted as a logo by medical organizations around the world (one example is the American Academy of Family Physicians), illustrates this duality with intriguing symbolism. Snake venom is a deadly poison. But in ancient China and India it was used to treat a variety of conditions, from opium addiction and skin cancers to problems with the liver. Today its medicinal uses include treating diseases affecting the immune system, such as MS and AIDS. And experimental studies with cobra venom have provided data that suggest it slows down the growth rate of certain cancers.

Another interesting characteristic of the snake is its ability to shed its skin. When a snake finishes molting, it appears newly hatched, just as a sick person who recovers from disease emerges rejuvenated. When we change our perspective and face the sun rather than the shadows, it's as if we are newly born: the body experiences our renewed love of life, and self-induced healing can result.

Historically, the staff carried by a traveling physician might have offered comfort and support to the onlooker, or it might have represented pain and death, depending on the condition of the patient and the skill of the practitioner. The serpent and staff combined into one symbol create a vivid reminder, for both practitioner and patient, of the positive and negative aspects of medical treatment.

As a physician-healer, I prefer to focus on symbols that reflect the power of love. We must remember as we care for each other that darkness, cold, and spiritual death exist only where there is no light, warmth, or love. The first image representative of healing that comes to my mind is that of the heart in an open palm. This symbol originated with the Shaker sect, who settled in the northeastern United States and followed a spiritual discipline of hard work and simplicity while devoting their lives to God. The hand represents charity, and the heart, compassion. The two combined imply a loving welcome and nonjudgmental acceptance, so the hand performs the act that the heart desires.

The therapeutic effect of compassion is infinite and immeasurable. A physician's genuine care for his or her patients enhances healing and can even eliminate the need for medical treatment or surgery. When a person receives caring attention, a live message enters his body at the cellular level. A young man dying of AIDS once shared with me his belief that "what is evil is not the disease, but to not respond with compassion to the person living with the disease."

Compassion doesn't have to come from outside sources. It can also be tapped from within. One of the imagery exercises I practice with my ECaP group involves turning fear or pain into a visual metaphor and working with that image. If you are struggling with fear or pain, try the following exercise. Imagine your fear or pain symbolized by a crying infant. Seated comfortably, close your eyes and imagine walking through your house, following the sound of that baby's heartrending sobs. As you enter a room, you find the child lying in its crib. Pick it up and hold it gently in your arms; rock and soothe the baby until it is comforted and stops crying. Then, carefully hold the baby away from your body. Be aware that it is not you, but that you can embrace it and learn from it. What lesson does this baby have to teach you?

This metaphor of the crying infant teaches you that your fear and pain provide an opportunity to walk into your shadows, attend to them, hold them, and soothe them. They should not be ignored or denied, but embraced and loved. The same exercise can be done when you are dreaming. Instead of running from the demon that appears, turn to face it in your dream; ask why it is there and what it wants of you.

It is no accident when one symbol appears in multiple countries, cultures, and eras and carries similar meanings in each despite the physical or chronological distance between occurrences. In modern science, for example, a triangle (which is also the Greek symbol called delta) symbolizes "a change." Weather forecasters will place a triangle in front of the letter T to signify a change of temperature, just as a nurse will draw one in front of the letters BP on a patient's chart to record a change in blood pressure.

The Alcoholics Anonymous logo is a triangle inside a circle, which represents that, for alcoholics to remain sober and enjoy long-term recovery, they must change their behavior and attitudes. Pyramids, built by ancient societies on both sides of the world, represented transformation, or change, from life to death, from this world to the other. Native Americans use triangles in their pottery, weavings, and jewelry to symbolize the portal through which spirit enters the newborn or returns to the ancestors.

Numbers too are symbols. All religions and cultures have, for example, seven days in a week, and the number seven represents a cycle of life. The number eight represents a new beginning. The number four represents completion or wholeness, just as the earth has four seasons and four directions.

Another kind of symbol consists of more than one image joined together in a metaphor, parable, or story. It illustrates a lesson or idea that people can easily grasp and experience. I began telling stories for two reasons. One of these reasons was beautifully illustrated by the author Isabel Allende during a lecture she gave several years ago and which I attended. When Allende related a Jewish proverb, its lesson really hit me, and I never forgot it. The proverb contains the question: What is truer than Truth? The answer is: A story.

I often spoke at Yale, trying to convince other doctors during grand rounds that the health improvements my ECaP patients were experiencing after joining the support group were genuine. When people heal their lives, I said, their disease heals, too. I cited various journals and articles, but the references I made to scientific data just opened the door to further arguments. Doctors would say to me, "I can't accept that." Some would even start yelling at me. "That's a poorly controlled experiment," they would tell me. Or they would say of whichever reference I cited: "That's not a good journal."

I even found that when I tried to do research, people would tell me, "What you're saying doesn't make sense, so we're not going to fund your research." Then others would say, "You've done no research, so why should we believe you?" I couldn't produce an acceptable answer in either case. People got angry at me and, finally, did research to prove I was wrong. When their results proved instead that my claims were correct, people in the medical profession began to open up to new possibilities.

One graduate student at Yale who was working on his master's thesis did a study involving the women with breast cancer in our support group. He came up with statistics that showed a significantly better survival rate among patients who embraced a mind-body-soul approach in a group that focused not on disease but on living life and taking responsibility for one's own recovery. It was impressive. When his professor saw these statistics derived from scientifically gathered data, he said, "That can't be true. You will have to change the control group."

You see, the student did the research and came up with something people didn't want to accept. His professor told him it couldn't be true, so he had to fix it. I explained to the student that people didn't have to be in my group to be survivors, that there are exceptional patients all over the world. To appease his professor, the student found a sufficient number of other individuals who did as well as those in our support group; this new data showed no significant difference between patients who embraced a mind-body-soul approach to their treatment and patients who didn't. Doctors accused me once again of lying, because "the research didn't prove anything."

What I learned was that if you got up in front of the same group of doctors and told a *story* about a patient, nobody walked out angry, since all I was doing was telling a story. It didn't threaten their belief system. It was an anecdote, a case history. But the story would have a significant effect. It would open the door and, a month later, if they had a "crazy" patient in their office, they'd say, "Hey, Siegel, you'll enjoy this." And then we'd start talking, and they'd begin to open their minds. Those stories became symbols of human potential for self-induced healing.

Instead of categorically disbelieving anything you can't consciously see, hear, or feel, at least open your mind and be *willing* to consider new ideas. Be like Jung and the great philosophers. Be like children and let your curiosity lead you into the wonder of life. Pay attention to symbols and archetypal characters and let them be your teachers.

In the next chapters, we will look at dreams and drawings and learn how symbols in them open the door to our inner wisdom. The mind is an incredibly powerful tool that can lead a person to survival or death, depending on the person's beliefs. What you believe is communicated to your body and affects how treatments, and the side effects of treatments, manifest within you.

DOCTOR'S R_x

Look through a magazine for archetypal characters and symbols. Perhaps you will find a doctor, a judge, a candle, a dollar bill, or a red rose.

Ask yourself whether its meaning is personal, universal, or perhaps both. Notice any emotions it evokes. Throughout the day, make a list of the symbols you consciously and unconsciously interact with. Notice what role they play in your thinking, emotions, behavior, and choices. Is one of the archetypes or symbols a frequent feature in your dreams? If so, what do you think it communicates to you?

Cut out a symbol that reminds you of a loving feeling, and tape it to your mirror or fridge as a love letter to yourself. Create shrines of love throughout your home, as I have in ours.

Chapter 3

THE POWER OF VISUALIZATION

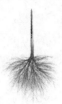

Each patient carries his own doctor inside him.

— ALBERT SCHWEITZER

I was not a typical surgeon, because I kept trying to help my patients in nontraditional ways. Although many doctors thought my methods were crazy, no one was against success, so if it worked for the patients, it became hospital policy. What I couldn't do, however, was convince the administrators to use the TV in patients' rooms to prepare them for surgery with guided imagery.

Mental imagery is not the same as just thinking about something. Analytical thinking happens mostly in regions on the left side of the brain, where language, planning, judgment, and numbers reign. Creative visualization, or mental imagery, is a process that engages mostly the right side, and other regions of the brain as well, since it involves using the visual, auditory, and olfactory senses, as well as memory, mood, emotions, and so on. The creative side of the brain can be used to prepare or train the mind and body for an experience, whether it involves learning a task, stabilizing mood, improving athletic performance, or healing a medical condition.

If you think about putting lemons on your shopping list, for example, the left side of your brain is activated when you are thinking, "I need to buy some lemons," and you notice that they cost $1.99 a pound. As an example of a creative visualization exercise, imagine holding a ripe, fresh lemon in your hand. Feel the waxy surface of the rind against your fingers, and smell the warm citrus aroma. Now imagine that you take a sharp knife and slice the lemon into quarters. Some of the juice sprays out and the lemony aroma becomes even stronger. Place one of the lemon quarters between your thumb and fingers and squeeze gently. Watch as the beads of juice rise up and trickle down the moist, plump flesh of the fruit. Raise the lemon to your mouth and let the juice trickle down to the back of your tongue.

By now you should be experiencing the lemon on an entirely different level. Your whole brain has engaged in the process. Your glands have begun to salivate and the bitterness of the lemon may have made you shudder or pucker your lips. Your body is responding as if you had tasted a real lemon. The process of visualization convinced your brain that the lemon was real.

Considering the immediate reaction your body had to the thought of a lemon experience, imagine what you could do by visualizing yourself going through surgery, chemotherapy, and radiation, and then healing without any negative side effects. I have witnessed this happening and heard amazing stories from hundreds of patients who used this wonderful mental tool to turn their fear of treatment into a powerful, loving, and healing experience.

Mental imagery is a technique that has long been used in the world of sports. Athletes have been coached to visualize a successful result of their movement such as a basketball shot or golf swing before they perform it, because when they do so they achieve better results. My friend who plays professional golf told me, "If my mind clearly pictures the ball landing where I want it to land, my body knows exactly what to do to produce that effect. I don't have to think about the details of grip, stance, and swing. I just imagine the end result and trust the rest of the job to the club and my swing."

Not until recent years could brain imaging, using technological aids such as fMRIs and PET scanners, measure and illustrate brain activity with great accuracy. These aids have become readily available and allow scientists to observe in real time what is actually happening in the brain. Alvaro Pascual-Leone's experiments at Harvard Medical School in the late 1990s involved volunteers learning a five-finger exercise on the piano.[1] One finding of his research was that volunteers who *imagined* doing the repetitive piano exercise experienced as much neural growth in the corresponding motor cortex of their brains as the volunteers who physically performed the exercise. Volunteers who practiced mental imagery fooled their brains into believing they were actually doing the physical exercise.

I had the opportunity to witness a similar phenomenon. One day before I performed a minor surgical procedure in my office, a patient and I got into an intense and interesting discussion. I picked up the scalpel while we were talking and made an incision. I noticed my nurse waving frantically at me. When she caught my attention she pointed at the syringe containing the local anesthetic which I had not used. I asked the patient how he was feeling, and he said he was fine, so I completed the surgery. I told him afterward that we had both been hypnotized by our discussion, and that I had not used any local anesthetic to numb the area of surgery. He was genuinely surprised. He had believed he was anesthetized, and so he felt no pain. Major surgery has also been done under hypnosis, and I have used hypnotherapists in the operating room as well.

My experience has also shown me that when people believed they were receiving radiation treatment, they had side effects and their tumors shrank, even though, because of a repair error, there was no radioactive material in the machine. You could say their belief became a form of self-hypnosis, or that they creatively visualized the radioactive material doing its job. No matter how you describe the process, their brains imagined that the treatment was actually taking place, and their bodies responded accordingly.

One woman wrote to me about her experience with a creative visualization technique she employed after she was diagnosed with lung cancer at age thirty-two.

> My neighbor's son was dying of bone cancer after being in remission for seven years. In spite of dealing with her own son's disease, this caring woman, when she heard about my diagnosis, took the time to tell me about your first book, *Love, Medicine & Miracles*. She described how you wrote about eating the cancer out with Pac-Men via the imagination. I visualized this every day and imagined myself running a marathon while my lungs remained pink and healthy. Thank God, when I went in for my repeat x-rays, it was gone, just gone. It took my doctor half an hour before he came and told me, because he had been running all over his office shouting the joyous news to everyone else!

While helping my patients to visualize their bodies eliminating disease, I have learned to avoid using language with negative connotations, such as *eating* or *killing* the cancer. For some patients the aggressive approach does not work. Instead of asking them to visualize Pac-Men, or animals, eating their cancer like a piece of meat, I help them to remove their disease in a loving way, such as by visualizing God's light melting a tumor that appears as a block of ice.

Sometimes patients ask me why oncologists recommend chemotherapy when they know this therapy can kill the patient. I explain to them that chemotherapy can, and does, save lives. The reality is that everyone dies, but if you elect to go on a healing journey, the key point to consider is: what labor pains are you willing to go through to rebirth yourself and make the pain worthwhile?

When a person is focused on the negative aspects of treatment, he needs to be empowered and given the chance to make his own decision about what is right for him, not simply to try to avoid dying. Patients should not focus solely on the disease; doing so empowers the enemy. This is why I emphasize so strongly the importance of a full partnership between patient and doctor. In that partnership, the patient has the advantage of learning about treatment options from a knowledgeable physician, and the doctor has the advantage of helping him make a decision the patient can live with and be comfortable with. I meet many people who prefer chemotherapy to being on a special diet, for example, because the diet is more of a problem to them than the medical treatment.

The mind is powerful. When you see treatment as a healing gift, you won't have all the side effects that can accompany that treatment. I ask people to draw themselves before they receive treatment; we can tell by such a drawing if the patient's image of treatment is negative. For example, I had a patient once who drew a picture of chemotherapy as the devil administering poison, so I knew there was a problem. In an instance like that, we can use visualization techniques to help the patient's subconscious turn the negative thought about chemo into a positive healing experience. If a patient can't turn her belief around, I recommend that she not choose to have it.

I can't say often enough that when you are facing a life-threatening illness like cancer, it is most important to find an oncologist you can communicate with openly, comfortably, and honestly. Most oncologists have never had chemo, and without firsthand knowledge of it they cannot fully understand the experience patients go through. The patient must be attended to with compassion, and his choices respected. If we retain our power as patients, the choice of physician and choice of treatment are ours to make. As I said, some people hate eating vegetables and prefer chemotherapy instead of a solely nutritional approach to treatment. Others want to let God heal them, and that's okay too. It is important that all patients are comfortable with their choices and do not become angry at themselves if things don't turn out as they had hoped.

To find a "good" doctor to treat your cancer, try to locate a "native" (that is, one who has had cancer), or one who has had a loved one affected by the disease. Also, choose a doctor who accepts criticism from patients, nurses, and family. Such doctors are the ones who see criticism as coaching and who learn from their mistakes. They don't make excuses or blame their patients. If you know someone who has been treated for cancer, ask what his doctor was like and if he recommends her. Ask a nurse which oncologist she would go to if she had cancer.

The potential for self-healing is built into you; a cut finger that heals by itself is a simple example of that. When you practice guided imagery, you are reprogramming your body. Guided imagery can help you do anything, so use it to see yourself becoming the person you want to be and doing the things you want to do. This is a powerful way to give your body whatever it needs to be well. Studies have shown that an actor's body chemistry changes according to whether the actor is given a comedy or a tragedy to perform. So mentally rehearse and practice visualization until you become the person you want to be.

Bobbie and I were down in Florida once, and we went to see a neurologist who is a friend. When we arrived, he was with a patient, so we sat in the waiting room. A few minutes later a nurse came in and said to me, "I'm putting a woman in the next room. She's going to the hospital shortly. I'm just letting you know so you won't make any noise, because she's in a lot of pain. She's had a migraine for over a week."

When the nurse left, I thought, "What is there to lose? Maybe I could help the woman with guided imagery or something." So I went into the next room and I asked, "What is the pain like?"

She said, "It feels like pressure."

If she had been my patient, my next question would have been:

"What is the pressure in your life?" But I said to her, "Let's look at the pressure in your head and in your life and relieve it." I did a little guided imagery exercise with her about relieving the pressure, and then I went out and sat down.

A few minutes later the bemused nurse returned to the waiting room. "She said her pain has completely disappeared and to tell you that the pressure was her marriage," the nurse told me. "After that, she left."

Our words create images, and our memories do the same thing. These images and memories are stored in our bodies, and when they are damaging they ultimately take their toll. So it is vitally important to feed our minds with healthy, positive images. It is very much the message of many spiritual teachers that we choose to see ourselves not as sick and disabled but as whole and filled with potential.

DOCTOR'S $\mathcal{R}_{x}$

If we are ill because of these intolerable images,
we get well because of imagination.

— JAMES HILLMAN

Find a comfortable position. Look up and let your eyelids close gently as you focus on your breathing, exhaling waste, inhaling inspiration. Allow a wave of peace to move through your body while you inspire life. When you feel ready, take a slow mental walk through your body. Find any wounds from the past. Love those areas; see them healing and becoming healthy and normal again. Picture your body doing what you want it to do. Continue mentally walking until you have journeyed throughout the whole body. Take time to enjoy the journey.

When you are finished, think about the places in your body where you now have, or have had, discomfort or other symptoms. Ask yourself what words you would use to describe your experience of the dis-ease or symptoms. Now think about relationships in your life that you could use the same words to describe. If a relationship or situation is affecting your health, drop the relationship or remove yourself from the situation. Think about what else in your life could be described the same way. When you pinpoint it, eliminate it from your life, and you will find relief from your symptoms too.

As you heal your life, your internal chemistry changes and your body benefits. Find the harmony and rhythm that are authentic for you, instead of accepting the ones imposed by others. Don't be afraid to imagine your ideal self; your body has the potential to create whatever you visualize. And when your health is not the issue, see how love can heal your life and cure your disease.

Chapter 4

DREAMS: THE BRAIN'S CREATIVE WORKSHOP

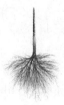

The dream is...by no means a dead thing that rustles like dry paper.
It is a living situation; it is like an animal with feelers,
or with many umbilical cords.

— CARL GUSTAV JUNG

At some time in our past, sleep was a dangerous undertaking. You'd lie down in your cave or shelter, and before many hours passed, a predator might come along. Many creatures do not sleep, or they sleep while standing, enabling them to wake and respond instantly to danger.

Adrian Morrison describes this paradox in his article "The Brain on Night Shift": "Although our brain waves are active during REM sleep, we are physically paralyzed..., not to mention unaware of our surroundings....We...are to all appearances defenseless, raising puzzling questions about REM sleep's role from the point of view of evolution."[1]

If the sleep state leaves us so vulnerable, why then do we do it?

What makes it worth the risk? Dreams provide creatures with a chance to practice survival behavior on a mental screen. We can encounter a monster or enemy in a dream when realistic practice is neither practical nor safe. There we can have the courage to confront and learn from what threatens us. When we're awake, we can apply this wisdom to our conscious life.

When animals sleep, the parts of their brains that activate visual and other senses are awake during dream states, even though their bodies are at rest. How often have you watched a sleeping dog twitch his paws as if chasing rabbits in his sleep? Athletes report that they play their sports in dreams in a sort of sleeping trial run, while writers have watched scenes of their works-in-progress unfold upon the dream's page. I have performed surgery in my dreams and learned from the experience both practically and emotionally.

I had a dream on the evening of Father's Day. In it I was a lottery winner, and when I awoke I realized it was a message about life as a lottery and how our five children and their families made me feel like a winner. As in this case, dreams can also confirm the things in our lives that are sources of strength and that are there to help us.

I believe the reason we sleep is not just to give our bodies a rest but also to allow a greater consciousness to speak to us through the symbols and stories of our dreams. I have had many dreams and experiences that have become personal guides and made me think about my life and actions and about creation as a whole. I have come to accept that, first, there was consciousness and consciousness was with God... and consciousness was God, because God speaks in dreams and images — the universal language.

Dreams and drawings contain information about your past, present, and the future you are unconsciously creating. I have had patients do drawings that included places and events that, as it turned out, were in their future. One drawing showed where a patient would die in an accident, and another patient's drawing had specific details showing what her operation room would look like (see fig. 22 in the insert), even though the patients had never been to those places before.

In chapter 3 we discussed creative visualization. While listening to an example of guided imagery on a CD or one given by a workshop facilitator, we leave worries and responsibilities behind. The guide's voice encourages us to go on a journey led by our intuition and imagination. Letting go of our conscious ego-mind, we enter a relaxed, safe, and creative realm where body and psyche merge. In the world of guided visualization, we are able to form bridges to the loving, peaceful energy that resides within us and that nurtures, heals, and promotes well-being.

When we dream, we go through a similar process, but instead of following the voice of another person, we become our own facilitator of imagery. The dream is our connection to our subconscious guide, our soul, our greater self.

The language of dreams is mostly pictorial, often symbolic, utilizing all of our senses and emotions. The stranger the images are, the more likely our subconscious wants us to pay attention. Dream images are all aspects of various parts of the dreamer. Often when you describe what was in your dream, you realize what it represents in your life or body.

For example, if you are under great stress from relentless challenges during the day, you might have a dream in which you are chased by an angry crowd. With feet too heavy to run, you flap your arms as hard as you can until your body miraculously rises above the clawing, outstretched hands of the people in that crowd. Flight seems the most natural thing to do. You soar higher and higher until you are above the clouds, and with a sense of great relief you feel like a child again, playing in the sky.

A dream such as this teaches us that we are capable of rising above our fears and worries. By doing so, it releases us and gives us the freedom to be ourselves and know that we can live in the joy of the moment. This dream experience of feeling like a child at play may also be a therapeutic message from an inner guide telling us to take a day off, walk on the beach, or begin practicing meditation or yoga and quiet the turbulent inner pond until our reflection is visible.

Our dreams also alert us to dangers that our consciousness is unaware of, such as disease developing in the body. As I noted earlier, Carl Jung interpreted a patient's dream and correctly diagnosed a brain tumor. I have had similar experiences with my patients, finding many of their dreams useful in diagnosing physical conditions. When a patient comes in to see me and says, "My mammogram was normal, but my dream wasn't," I always respond with: "Okay, we'll do a biopsy." Over the years, I found that each time one of my patients' dreams told him or her something like that, the biopsy resulted in a diagnosis of cancer. I learned to respect patients' inner wisdom because it was always right. I know patients who had to see five doctors before one finally said okay and did a biopsy, which revealed cancer. I also know patients who died when they didn't follow their dream's warning, or when doctors didn't listen to them and the patient didn't persist and insist on having a biopsy.

Susan Hoffman shared her story in my last collection, *A Book of Miracles*. In her dream, a small-framed Asian woman with slender fingers touched the top of her right breast and said, "The cancer is right there." When Susan woke, she found a lump exactly in the spot where the woman in her dreams had touched her, so she went to her doctor and a biopsy was scheduled. Days later, Susan went to UCLA to have the biopsy. She wrote, "I was put into a room in which the doctors would come in and feel the tumor site. When they left, and I started to get dressed, an Asian doctor came rushing in to say she was in a hurry to get to surgery, touched my breast, and said, "Oh yeah, it's right there, the cancer's right there." Immediately Susan recognized that this doctor's hand was the one from her dream.[2]

Years ago, when I experienced bloody urine, my colleagues wanted me to immediately go and have it evaluated. I was very busy and didn't listen to their concerns or make an appointment to have it looked into.

That night I had a dream in which I was sitting in our cancer support group, and we were all introducing ourselves. When it was my turn, before I could say anything, everyone turned to me and said, "But you don't have cancer." So I knew I was okay, and I was. I did see a urologist and had the infection treated, but it was done without stress and fear because of my confidence in the dream.

One patient told his doctor about a dream he had in which a beaver dam kept obstructing the flow of a river. It caused him so much distress that he woke and could not get the dream out of his mind. He even told his doctor about it during a regular checkup. His doctor made the symbolic connection between rivers and arteries and immediately ordered tests to be done. These revealed that the man had an obstructed coronary artery, a condition that, left untreated, would have ended his life.

Some dreams prepare us for difficult news. Andrea Hurst felt trapped in an unhappy marriage with a partner whose abusive behavior left her feeling depressed, powerless, and with no place to turn. One night she dreamt that she was walking with a crowd of people who were carrying signs and demonstrating about something that was really important to fight for. She grew afraid of the surging mass and pulled off to the side, but she knew she had to make a choice to either fight along with them or give in. She was aware that the stakes were high. Summoning all her courage, she decided to fight and rejoined the demonstration.

Soon after the disturbingly vivid dream, Andrea was diagnosed with breast cancer. At first she was tempted to surrender, but she remembered the dream and decided not to give up on herself. Andrea agreed to have surgery. She got hold of my books and tapes and maintained a daily dialogue with God. "As soon as I realized that being trapped was not my reality, but rather my outlook, I gained a sense of power back and my outlook changed," she later told me. "I no longer felt like a victim of circumstances. The dream illustrated that I could do what was right for me, and it gave me the courage to leave the marriage.

Once I left, I created a peaceful, loving environment for myself — one that supported the positive effects of my surgery and treatment."

Another woman felt conflicted about the therapy that she and her doctor had decided on. When she dreamt about a white cat who revealed its name was Miracle, and who told her what treatment was best for her, she wrote it all down and got her doctor to follow Miracle's advice. She listened to her inner voice, the wisdom of her dream, and years later she was alive, healthy, and well.

Many times I met patients who had seen anatomical structures in their dreams, although they had no conscious knowledge of what these structures look like in the body. One woman refused surgery to remove her thymus gland as treatment for myasthenia gravis. After many weeks of deteriorating health, she had a dream about a gray object with fingerlike extensions growing into her body. She asked her doctor what a normal thymus looked like, and when he described it she realized hers was not normal, so she agreed to have the surgery. When she woke, she asked her doctor to describe what the diseased thymus had looked like. He held up his hand, curled it and said, "It looked like this, with finger-like extensions." Her thymus contained a malignant growth, and her dream had accurately portrayed it.

Just as the artist loses awareness of the world as he paints on his canvas, during the dream state our analytical consciousness is temporarily set aside, preventing ego interference. Instead of interrupting our dream with a censoring thought, such as "This is ridiculous; don't pay attention to this," we sit and observe while watching the movie unfold on the screen. Swept into the dream world, we experience acute sensations, desires, and knowledge by means of the dream's settings, actions, sounds, sights, smells, and even tastes.

Cathy Thayer was a teacher of twenty-eight special-needs children. She enjoyed her work and was devoted to her students, but the mental, physical, and emotional demands she took upon herself had been seriously affecting her health. At the end of her first year of teaching, Cathy was diagnosed with breast cancer. She refused to give up on her students, and despite undergoing chemotherapy and follow-up treatments over the next five years, she continued to teach.

One morning Cathy woke feeling exhausted and deeply disturbed. She had dreamt that hundreds of people had been camping on her front lawn. Paying no attention to her pleas for peace and quiet, the campers had made bonfires with her garden furniture, scattered garbage, used the lawn as a toilet, and created nonstop noise. "The campers crossed all my boundaries and had no respect for me as a person," Cathy told me. "They acted as if I were there solely to provide for them. Catering to their needs was ruining my life."

After the dream recurred several times, alerting her that she had not resolved the problem, Cathy realized her subconscious was trying to show her what the stress of special-needs teaching was doing to her. "I had not been listening to my body, so my subconscious decided to shake my shoulders and scream, 'Wake up! Your job is killing you!' That's when I made the decision to quit teaching full-time. Since then my health has been much better; the cancer is gone, and the dream has not returned."

Many years ago one of my patients was facing a decision about her treatment. She talked about a dream in which she had to choose between taking the elevator or the staircase. She chose the staircase. After discussing it with me, she came to the realization that her dream showed she was determined to rely on herself rather than use mechanical methods of getting well. While she knew the stairs were an uphill climb, she felt much better about choosing methods that stemmed from her own inner wisdom and strength.

Sometimes dreams save lives when doctors miss vital information. Ruth was being treated with medication for pain in her lower abdomen. One night she dreamt the same dream four times, each recurrence after waking and falling asleep again. In her dream, a very gentle man was holding a knife in a nonthreatening way over the left side of her lower abdomen. When she finally realized that the dream was telling her she needed an operation, she was able to sleep without disturbance. The next day she made an appointment with her gynecologist. She asked the surgeon to remove her left tube and ovary and her uterus. After the surgery, the pathology report came back showing she'd had a fast-growing tumor on the left side of her uterus.

Dreams can also open the door to messages of love, comfort, and approval, messages that cross the physical barriers erected by our consciousness, intellect, or ego. These dreams often acknowledge that the path we are on is the correct path, or they may show us a source of strength, in this way supporting and encouraging us on our journey. When your intuitive side knows the right way at a deep level, it participates with your consciousness, and the direction of your life becomes clear.

Shortly after starting the cancer support groups, I wondered if I did it for unhealthy reasons related to my fear of cancer and death. That night I had a dream in which I was a passenger in a car that went off a cliff; everyone else was screaming, but I was calm with the thought of death as a result. I awoke knowing fear was not my issue. Just as I became a surgeon to fix things and not because I enjoy cutting people up, my dream confirmed I was running the group for healthy reasons.

After her release from a psychiatric hospital following a nearly successful suicide attempt, Kelly began working through a twelve-step recovery program to address drug and alcohol addiction. In her letter to me she described a dream that portrayed strength and wisdom with symbols that were meaningful to her.

So much of my early recovery was shrouded by a barrage of emotions and fear that never seemed to leave me. But the night I reached six months of sobriety, I had a dream that gave me a new awareness.

I found myself staring into the eyes of a lion that looked as if he had swallowed the sun, such intense light emanated from them. The lion was surrounded by swirling deep-blue water, and beneath the surface his front right paw was shackled. A small lion cub, precious and innocent, was chained to the adult lion, and I felt a strong desire to protect it. Despite my fear, I was in awe of the lion's strength and raw power. I was terrified and trembling, but I managed to release the cub, all the while giving the adult lion as wide a berth as possible.

Once the cub was free, I turned back to look at that magnificent beast of light and gold, and it reminded me how close I had come to the brink of losing everything — losing myself. I had been so ashamed because I had accomplished nothing with my life and had tried to throw my life away. But now I was facing my fears and emotions without the use of chemicals. I was walking the journey through acceptance, willingness, and faith. Saving the lion cub proved my courage and strengthened my commitment. The dream made me see how much I have accomplished in six months. Now I have nothing to be ashamed of and everything to love about myself.

The process of restructuring your life, of becoming an authentic person, requires that you see yourself as dynamic, ever changing, and *becoming*. I always like to remember that graduations are commencements, and that the Bible ends in a revelation, not a conclusion. Our dreams, such as Kelly's lion, illustrate this aspect, and they encourage us to keep striving. It is the process of living that is important, that we all struggle with, not the end product or the result. Life is a journey. Rather than search for meaning in life, we bring meaning to our lives by how we love ourselves and how we love the world.

Sometimes dreams help us to let go of things from our past that are no longer useful. When Jean was a child, her mother died from breast cancer that had metastasized to her bones. Jean received no counseling or supportive help from the adults in her life, and she was discouraged from expressing her grief after her mother died. Later, in her adult years, Jean suffered from chronic panic attacks that left her paralyzed with fear and unable to drive. Since she was the only person in the family who *could* drive, it was a difficult problem that affected everyone in her family.

Jean decided to attend a spiritual retreat that was being held in a place where she had never been before. One week before the event, she dreamt that she went to a large hotel that overlooked a beautiful garden. A long staircase from the main lobby led to bedrooms above, and classes took place in rooms on the ground floor. A nurse came down the stairs and asked Jean if she wanted to see her mother, who had secretly been living in the hotel for all those years. Gripped with hope, fear, and shock, Jean walked out to the garden, unsure about meeting her mother again. Losing her the first time had been too painful. Finally she agreed to a reunion, and the nurse went to get her mother. But the nurse returned alone and announced that Jean's mom had just died. No reunion could happen. Jean woke up from the dream sobbing tears that she had withheld as a child.

A week later, Jean arrived at the spiritual retreat only to discover that the hotel was the same as the one in her dream. At first she wanted to turn and run, but her curiosity convinced her to stay. On the third day of the retreat, Jean went into the garden during a break. A voice seemed to come from nowhere, telling her that for all those years, she had been holding on to her grief only because it was the last thing that connected her to her mother. Jean feared that if she let go of the grief there would be nothing left but a void. "It is okay to let go," said the voice. "You have nothing to fear. You are never, ever alone, for I am with you."

Jean did not tell anyone at the retreat about her experience. Later that day, she was given a slip of paper by the retreat facilitator. On it was printed the following biblical quote: *Fear not, for I am with you.* Since then, Jean has not had another panic attack. Her dream became her connection to the higher spirit who loved her and healed her from within.

Hearing a voice does not mean you are going crazy. I have heard voices many times, and they have always helped me to heal my life and emotions.

Claire Sylvia, the exceptional patient I first discussed in the introduction, had vivid dreams after her heart-lung transplant. Through her dreams after the surgery, she began to know the donor and to trust what she intuitively knew was real communication with his spirit. While this phenomenon has not been recorded by the majority of transplant recipients, many have claimed that they had postoperative memories, or gained new preferences, that originated with their organ donors. Claire was surprised when she suddenly wanted to drink beer, eat chicken nuggets, and ride a motorcycle. Some organ recipients have also, like Claire, reported dreams involving the donor.

Claire described the "most unforgettable dream of my life" in her book, *A Change of Heart*. In the dream she was outdoors with a slender young man, and they enjoyed being together. When it was time for her to leave, they kissed. She writes, "As we kiss, I inhale him into me. It feels like the deepest breath I've ever taken, and I know that [he] will be with me forever."[3]

The young man appeared in many more of Claire's dreams and, over the years, showed her things that helped her to locate the donor's family and to confirm that the visual impressions and memories of her dream visitor were indeed those of the young man whose heart and lungs had given her body life.

Our minds and bodies are in constant communication with each other, and most of this happens at the level of unconsciousness. Because of this, I often advise patients to start recording their dreams. The body cannot communicate except through symbols, and while the symbolic imagery in dreams may be difficult to understand at first, with practice and guidance we can learn to interpret our dreams. By using imagery and recording our dreams, we unlock and open the treasure chest of the unconscious.

Dr. Gillian Holloway offers a simple five-step plan for gathering and interpreting dreams in her book, *Dreaming Insights*. She encourages the dream journalist, before going to sleep, to enter the date on his journal page, write a short description of that day's events, and follow with a question that he would like his dream to answer. Holloway recommends that, in the morning when writing down the dream, the writer use present tense, which will help him to reenter the dream.[4]

One reader who tried this method wrote to me saying that, for the first time, she was able to remember not just one dream but three. Writing down and analyzing the progression of the three dreams upon waking gave her valuable insight.

> Before I went to bed I was troubled by an undesired relationship split, and I asked my dreams to help me understand what I needed to learn from this. As I slept, I thought I was awake, and I felt a presence beside me observing the dreams. After each one, I woke and I wrote down a few key words with some difficulty while in my state of half sleep. In the morning, I remembered all three dreams in vivid Technicolor and was able to write coherently about what I had seen and how I felt in each dream.
>
> When I looked at the symbolic objects and actions in the dreams, phrases popped into my head, so I wrote them down as well. In one scene I was walking on a path and came to a place where it split. On the right, I saw a giant fir tree, its branches covered with thousands of luscious new green shoots. It was so beautiful that I chose to enter that path. A line from Robert Frost's poem popped into my mind, about two roads diverging in a yellow wood, as well as the significance of the green shoots, which promised abundance and life if I followed this path.
>
> When I finished writing all this down, I felt as if scattered pieces of a jigsaw had been joined together, and I was able to see and understand the bigger picture. I realized exactly what I needed to learn from the recent disturbing events, and I felt at peace in my new circumstances. Everything is just as it was meant to be, and it is all good. I'm looking forward now to using my dream journal as a creative and fun tool for growth.

DOCTOR'S R_x

A dream that is not interpreted is like a letter that is not read.

— THE TALMUD

Keep a loose-leaf notebook and pen by your bedside. After you wake, record your dreams in as much detail as you can. Write every little thing you remember, even if it doesn't seem important. Don't worry about the quality of the writing; just get the dream down on paper. Include the feelings you experienced during the dream and those that lingered upon waking. When you have finished writing, be aware of recurrent themes, patterns, symbolic images, and signs. Make notes in the margins and underline things that stand out. Do this for one week. You may want to discuss what you recorded with a dream partner or counselor. Did anything previously hidden become clear to you? Did your partner pick up on things that you missed?

Chapter 5

DRAWINGS: WHEN CONSCIOUS AND UNCONSCIOUS DISAGREE

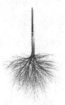

Art is when you hear a knocking from your soul — and you answer.

— TERRI GUILLEMETS

When we realize that images and symbols from dreams are a dialogue between our psychic or somatic intelligence and our conscious mind, it becomes easy to see that drawings too may be a form of communication with the collective consciousness and our greater self. I was introduced to spontaneous drawings at a workshop facilitated by Elisabeth Kübler-Ross in the late 1970s. Kübler-Ross, a psychiatrist, Jungian, and author of *On Death and Dying*, devoted her life to improving medical professionals' understanding of death as a growth process that involves stages of adjustment (denial, anger, bargaining, depression, and acceptance), and she beneficially influenced the hospice concept and care of terminally ill patients.[1]

One of Kübler-Ross's therapeutic tools for opening communication between the dying patient and the people involved in that patient's care was the use of spontaneous drawings. Drawings helped to reveal emotional issues that patients and family members had not felt comfortable discussing, and these drawings provided another means of identifying unfinished business before the death happened.

Having learned about the significance of dreams, and having witnessed the positive effects of guided visualization, I was excited to attend the Kübler-Ross workshop, meet Elisabeth, and gain a new Jungian surgical tool to share with my patients.

Throughout the weekend, a mixture of patients and health care professionals were given the opportunity to share their emotions and life experiences and create drawings. These workshops were followed by sessions in which Elisabeth introduced and practiced the interpretation techniques she used.

I was surprised by the authenticity of what Elisabeth revealed to me from my drawings alone — things I had been consciously unaware of, and which she brought to light through her questions and observations. For example, I chose to draw an outdoor scene depicting a snowcapped mountain and, below it, a pond with a fish jumping out of the water.

When Elisabeth studied my picture, her first question was: "What are you covering up?"

"What do you mean?" I asked. I thought my picture revealed how much I value the peace and beauty of nature. She then pointed to the snow.

"You used a white crayon on white paper. Putting white on white was unnecessary; you added a layer that suggests you are covering something up. You also drew a fish — a spiritual symbol — but it's a fish out of water."

A year before the workshop, I had shaved my head. Many thought I did it in support of my cancer patients, but it was simply an inner desire I couldn't resist. I had no idea what my motivation had been until that day in the workshop. I suddenly realized I had been keeping a lid on my feelings, as well as on my spirituality, in order to protect myself from the pain I felt at being unable to fix and cure all my patients. Cutting my hair had been a symbolic attempt to remove the lid, but I needed to uncover more than skin.

The snowcapped peak and jumping fish illustrated my feelings of separation from my spiritual, loving self, just as my shaved head was not about revealing skin but was a symbolic act, like that of a monk who uncovers his head as a symbol of uncovering his spirituality. Once I understood that, I found inner peace, and Elisabeth became my guide and teacher.

The insights I gathered at the workshop confirmed that communication was happening between my conscious and subconscious through the drawings. What excited me as a physician, however, was what I observed in the drawings of the people attending. Not only were psychological aspects of their lives reflected in their sketches, but also many of them drew anatomically correct aspects of their bodies and diseases without even realizing they had done so. Being a surgeon, I recognized the anatomical structures that patients and psychologists often had little or no knowledge of. Because of the physical and psychological aspects of the drawings, I was convinced that the practice would create a valuable means of communication between patients, physicians, and other people involved in the patients' care. I went back to my office and the hospital armed with a box of crayons, my new surgeon's tools.

Many physicians refused to believe what I was telling them; it was not something they had been exposed to during their training. How to teach your patients to induce self-healing is not a topic taught in medical school. So until the physicians experienced what I had observed and participated in, they refused to accept it.

Spontaneous drawings are an excellent resource for prevention, diagnosis, prognosis, and treatment of an illness. Rather than *replace* medical interventions, the drawings become an *additional resource* and enhance the physician's skill. With insight into the patient derived from the wisdom of the subconscious, both physician and patient can make better therapeutic decisions. People thought I was crazy when I asked my patients to create drawings before making any treatment recommendations or decisions, but every time patients got over their fear about not being artists and just drew, the drawings proved to be powerful guides that we could not afford to ignore.

Doctors are not trained in how to speak to people, so when they say, "We're giving you chemotherapy and here are the side effects...," they don't precede it with: "This will cure you or prolong your life." It's like the TV ads: after they tell you a pill is good for you, they say it might give you a heart attack, make your liver fail, sterilize you, make your hair fall out, or kill you. As scary as the ends of the ads are, at least they start with the benefits of a drug before they tell you the possible side effects. What patients hear from doctors about side effects is designed so the hospital and doctor won't get sued. The hospital and doctor don't think about the effect words from an authority figure have on a patient's feelings and decision-making process. That's why I always start out with: "This can make you well and add years to your life" or "It can cure you. There are some side effects, but they don't happen to everybody." I call it "deceiving" people into health. I slant the information for their benefit, accentuating the positive, because people can be talked into health or illness.

One man who came to see me insisted that he did not want chemotherapy even though it was the recommended treatment for his cancer. He was unable to express the reason for his concerns, but I was certain I knew what the problem was. He was afraid of the side effects because of what his physician had said. I asked this man to draw a picture of the recommended treatment (fig. 18). He drew the chemotherapy as yellow fluid running into him, not all over his body and making him sick, but going directly to the cancer. It was coming from the east and looked like sunlight — a positive sign of energy. On the left side of the page, one of his white cells was riding a horse and piercing the cancer. I explained to him that his intuition was saying chemotherapy was the right treatment for him and it was going to work.

When you connect with a patient's inner wisdom, he recognizes that it's coming not from the doctor but from within himself, and suddenly the lightbulb goes on; that moment of enlightenment occurs, and you can see it in his face. At that point, I said to him, "Go and get the chemotherapy; it's the right thing for you to do." His attitude had changed, and he was able to accept the recommended treatment. He approached his chemotherapy treatment with hope and confidence, and it turned out to be the right choice.

Another patient drew an illustration of his kitchen with everyone in his family shown upside down, as if they were standing on their heads. I asked him to explain what was going on, and he said he had chosen to treat his cancer with a macrobiotic diet instead of chemotherapy. "The kids don't eat with me anymore. My wife hates preparing it, and I don't like eating it. I'd rather have chemotherapy." Until that drawing revealed his growing sense of sadness about the diet undermining his family relationships and his feelings of loss at not being able to share meals with them, he had been unable to voice his unhappiness about his decision not to have chemotherapy.

"You don't have to treat your cancer with vegetables," I said. "You can still elect to have chemotherapy and treat the cancer that way." His eyes lit up and he looked happy for the first time since he entered my office. Seeing his true feelings illustrated on paper motivated him to choose what his instinct felt was right for him, and he had the chemotherapy treatment.

When the subconscious and conscious minds, a patient's two sources of wisdom, are in conflict about a treatment, the patient will inevitably suffer more problems and side effects. You may have two patients with the same cancer getting the same treatment. But when one patient draws the operating room, and all you can see is him alone, lying on the operating table, this patient will have more trouble related to pain and postoperative side effects (fig. 57). When the other patient draws an unmasked surgeon holding her with music, love, God, and rainbows, she will awaken from surgery sore but free of major pain or side effects, and she will recover rapidly (fig. 58).

Patients' unexpressed fear of treatment can often be identified by the images in their drawings. When a patient draws a negative image such as her chemotherapy syringe filled with black liquid (fig. 52), I have her visualize the same therapy with a positive result, one that is free of side effects. I created a CD called *Getting Ready* that helps patients to adopt positive thoughts and beautiful images related to their treatment. These become autohypnotic and help patients make the right decision and prepare their bodies to expect a positive result no matter what that treatment is. After a week or so, the patient's next drawing will look different compared to the original version, and it will confirm that the conflict between intellect and intuition has been resolved to the benefit of that patient. Treatment can go ahead then with few or no side effects and will produce better results. If a patient cannot visualize a positive result, I try to help him or her clarify the difference between trying not to die and choosing what is right for him or her.

In earlier chapters, we discussed the power of creative visualization to stimulate the immune system's reaction to chemotherapy and cancer. When a patient draws his treatment and shows white blood cells eliminating the cancer (fig. 59), or a patient draws beams of golden light streaming through her body (fig. 58), this patient is utilizing God-given tools for self-induced healing. Whatever we imagine, and what we focus on, sends a message to our body, so when we draw healing images our body follows through. After guided visualization, if a patient's drawings show positive symbols and imagery (fig. 64), I have no worries about the outcome of her treatment. Such people have a remarkable recovery record, and I know this patient will be okay.

Disease often strikes where the body has stored painful memories of the past. A patient's inner wisdom recognizes that these memories need to be acknowledged in order to heal. Psychologist and author Alice Miller says, "The truth about our childhood is stored up in our body, and someday the body will present its bill ... until we stop evading the truth."[2] In *Breaking Down the Wall of Silence*, she says, "Your real felt feelings will never kill you; they will help you find direction. Only the unfelt yet powerful emotions and needs, the feared and banished ones, can kill us.... Therapists were surprised to see that once patients could...take their unwanted emotions seriously and develop them into a direct and healthy language, full recovery was possible."[3]

Pain helps us to identify and define ourselves; when we realize that, and work with it, all pain becomes labor pain, or growing pains. When spontaneous drawings bring up old hurts from the past, they make it possible to deal with psychic wounds that have the potential to become physical disease. And labor pains are worthwhile when we give birth to our true selves.

Dr. Caroline Thomas, a professor and psychiatrist at Johns Hopkins Medical School, had medical students fill out a personality profile and draw a picture of themselves as part of a long-term study that continued to follow them after they left medical school and that collects data to this day. Years later Thomas looked at the medical histories and found that specific aspects of their original drawings and personality profiles significantly correlated with diseases the students experienced after medical school, and they also correlated with the parts of the body that were affected. This stimulated further medical research into predicting with some accuracy what diseases people are likely to have later in life, and in what part of the body, based on personality profiling. One of the factors for predicting cancer turned out to be a profile that reported a low level of closeness to parents.[4]

Children in particular are unprepared to deal with physical or emotional trauma when it happens, and they are vulnerable to whatever their adult authority figures impose at the time. If caring adults do not help them deal with trauma, children will resort to a coping mechanism that leads them to store the feelings and memories of events in their subconscious mind and body, to be dealt with at a later time or never resolved. Seeds of anxiety, grief, fear, abandonment, and other emotions plant themselves in parts of the body and lie dormant until years later, when the immune system is challenged by the stress of grief or another traumatic event. It is then that these seeds can manifest into conditions such as cancer, heart disease, respiratory or digestive ill-ness, allergies, and more. These potential illnesses are often revealed in patients' drawings — and not just their own potential illnesses but also those of other family members.

I would be concerned about a mother's drawing of her family in which her son carries an empty oval object that resembles the hole in the nearby tree trunk — a symbol of the family's situation surround-ing the mother's cancer (fig. 61). This patient's drawing shows her son at the end of the line, not connected to anyone. The boy's life is like the empty vessel under his arm. Analyzing a drawing like this enables the parents not to feel criticized but to see their son's unexpressed loneliness and grief, even when it is expressed intuitively in the mother's drawing. The father needs to be connected to the mother, and the family to each other; together they can take whatever action is needed to help the boy feel loved and supported as the family members go through the ordeal.

Connections between significant or traumatic memories and one's present state of health are often revealed in the drawings. Once they are made visible, the person can give much-needed attention to the past affliction and the soul. This is never about blaming the patient, but about how our emotions create our internal chemistry and affect our genes and health.

A good example of this is a nonbelieving reporter who asked me for an interview. Right away I could see that this very intellectual per-son lived in her head, not her heart. I realized it wasn't going to be a pleasant interview, so I had to do something to change her perspec-tive right at the start. I said to her, "While I finish up with the last two patients, please draw a picture of yourself." She agreed to do so, and when she handed me her drawing, I saw a figure with a big head, so I realized my diagnosis of her attitude was correct (fig. 45). Her drawing also contained a clock with one hand pointing at twelve.

The safest question for me to ask her would have been: Why is twelve important to you? She might have responded, "Twelve months ago my house burned down." But I wanted to really shake her up, so I took a chance and, pointing to the clock, asked, "What happened when you were twelve years old?"

"It means I don't like deadlines."

"But there's only one hand on the clock. What happened when you were twelve years old?"

She burst into tears and told me that at twelve years of age she had been abused. That's the part that always impresses me — numbers in drawings are no accident. From that moment on, it was a different interview. The reporter understood that her inner wisdom was telling her to pay attention to the feelings of the traumatized inner child, to stop hiding from the memory by living in her head, and to seek therapeutic help.

Drawings not only connect aspects of mind and body, but they also integrate patients' lives outside the clinical arena with somatic aspects of their diseases. A doctor sent me a drawing by a patient who was having pelvic problems. Despite giving her various treatments, no one had been able to relieve her symptoms. Her drawing revealed a heart, like a valentine heart, with a large crack in it and twenty drops of blood dripping from the heart. I told him to ask her what happened when she was twenty, and her answer revealed sexual abuse at the age of twenty as the etiology of her problem. Numbers are not always about one's age; she could have answered that twenty months ago something happened. When she received counseling for the trauma, her symptoms were relieved.

Other drawings have identified the causes of symptoms. One girl's mother was distraught, believing that her child's enlarged cervical lymph nodes were a sign that her daughter had a lymphoma, a disease that ran in her family. When the woman brought her in to be examined, she also brought two of the child's drawings. In one picture the girl had drawn herself with a swollen neck and face, and in the other she drew a cat with large front claws. I told the mother not to worry, that her daughter had cat scratch fever. Tests and a biopsy revealed this to be the correct diagnosis.

When we expose the unconscious and reveal the inner truth,

disharmony between individuals, families, and health care professionals ceases. No longer do intellect and intuition remain in conflict, so
true healing can occur. There may be physicians who will say, "Who
has time for this?" My answer is that you save time by using drawings.
When a child with cancer tells me she is not getting enough time from
her family, I can talk to six people in her family and try to clarify the
issue, or I can ask her to draw a picture of the family.

One child with cancer drew her family seated on a couch. At the end
of the couch she left an empty space for one more person, but she drew
herself seated on a chair at the other side of the room. Her parents' arms
were either wrapped around her siblings or protecting themselves, and
they were physically distant from their sick daughter (fig. 62).

I didn't need to spend an hour explaining to the parents that their
daughter was feeling abandoned, for one look at the picture said it all.
Once they understood their daughter's viewpoint, they were able to
express how their fear of losing her had resulted in their withdraw-
ing emotionally as a coping mechanism and so they could be strong
for their other children. The fact that the sick girl drew herself in the
spiritual color purple also said to me that she knew she was going to die
of the cancer.

The picture played a significant role in changing the parents'
behavior. They began talking with each other more about their feelings, and they gave their daughter the extra attention and loving support she needed. Not only did it help the child through her ordeal, but
also the whole family grew closer before she died. When we allow spirit
and symbol to serve life, we can be unique guides and life coaches for
those we care for and about. We can be aware of the truth and not see a
person's death as a failure. And we can allow ourselves to continue our
lives free of guilt, as this child's parents were able to do.

METHOD AND THEORY

To create your own drawings or to facilitate the work of others, you
need not be an artist or therapist. All you need is some plain white paper

and a box of crayons or colored pencils. You must have all the colors of the rainbow available for use, plus black, white, and brown, since every color has meaning associated with it.

I avoid telling people what to draw, because I want their unconscious, inner wisdom to have the freedom to create a drawing that reveals unasked questions and unspoken desires. But when cancer or another disease is the situation or theme, I ask the person to draw a picture of himself that shows his disease and treatment, with his white blood cells eliminating the disease. I avoid using words that suggest killing or a warlike approach, as I am interested in helping people to heal their lives and bodies, not focus on their enemy. I may also ask a person to draw a self-portrait, an outdoor scene, or his home and family.

You can draw a picture that relates to a decision you have to make, such as a job choice, the person you will marry, or upcoming surgery. I encourage people to include any images, objects, and symbols that pop into mind while they are working on their drawings. Children are not self-critical as they work, but adults need to be told there is no wrong way to draw the picture; this is necessary to eliminate their fear that they and their drawings will be judged and found wanting.

The evaluator's first step is to write down her immediate overall impression and identify any feelings evoked by the picture, such as isolation, anger, sadness, or joy. The next step is to see what is in the picture (people, objects, movement and direction of movement, body size, and so on). Notice what is missing (such as hands or feet) and what is odd about the drawing, as well as any accidents or errors (such as lines that cross over a person). The evaluator should pay attention to the colors used, to their intensity and shade, to available colors that were not used, and to any odd color choices (such as a purple sun). She should also pay attention to numbers and count recurring objects. In a picture that has multiple themes and elements, the evaluator can make note of which quadrants each symbol or image is in. She should observe how completely the drawing fills the page and check to see if the artist also drew on the other side of the paper.

Before analysis begins, the artist should be available to discuss the drawing with the evaluator and answer questions related to it. To interpret it correctly, we need to know why the person drew what he did. For instance, a child handed me a drawing done entirely in black crayon, and I was worried about him until he said, "I have two older brothers. That's the only crayon I ever get."

The evaluator must understand that she represents an authority figure. If she bases her interpretation of the drawing only on her own understanding and beliefs, she may misinterpret it or may appear to criticize it — and both of these can cause harm. The drawing is not meant to be read like a horoscope, but should be used as a therapeutic tool for discussion with the artist so that correct interpretations and choices can be made.

As an example of an evaluation that needs clarification, consider a patient's drawing of his treatment that includes a black cat walking across the floor. Let's say that, to the evaluator, the cat suggests something negative, a threat, when in reality the patient has a black cat and his subconscious is expressing the idea that the cat's presence during treatment would be something positive, a source of comfort and love. Instead of revealing an emotional problem or threat, the black cat in this drawing represents an important aspect of the patient's recovery needs.

The color purple, a spiritual color, may reveal a coming transition from physical body to spirit through an appropriate symbol, such as a purple butterfly going up into the sky. But a patient who draws himself wearing purple may not be predicting his own death. For him purple might represent his spiritual nature. Or it may be the color of his favorite basketball team, and so may signify a victory over his disease, one that will enable him to attend and enjoy many more games. It is essential, then, that whoever is guiding the artist in the interpretation of his drawing be open-minded and nonjudgmental during the dialogue between them, for the artist is the expert in analyzing the meaning of what has been drawn. The therapist is there only to help bring out the hidden meaning, as one would do with someone else's dream.

Past, present, and future may all be represented in a person's drawing. At some level of consciousness, we are aware of the future because, as Jung said, we unconsciously create our future far in advance. This awareness extends to important life changes and events, as well as to our upcoming death, whether it will be due to an accident or a disease.

One drawing, done by a woman with cancer, showed her husband flying a purple kite. I realized she was saying that she was ready to go and that he wasn't able to let go of her because she took care of everything. When I suggested this to her, she went to him and said, "I'll train you." Six months later he told her he cut the string, and she responded, "I'll die Thursday when the kids get here from California." And she did.

I asked one woman to draw a picture, and she drew a gravestone with three green shrubs planted in front of it. To the left, soil was piled beside an empty grave. Green is the color of life, so it seemed to suggest that in the face of death she chose to live instead. How long do you think she lived? She was interred in the grave nearly three years to the day after she drew this picture (fig. 24).

Drawings can simply relate to what is happening now in the artist's life, but those that contain multiple objects or complex content can often be divided into quadrants where the past, present, and future are revealed, as on a grid.

The center of the drawing represents what is centrally significant to the artist, as in the drawing of the woman who represented her breast cancer with two sails on a boat (fig. 12). The upper right quadrant of a picture represents the present, or the "here and now" (see fig. 19), where the artist, diagnosed with cancer, shows his children as birds in the top right corner. Downward-pointing wings reveal their current grief about the situation and their inability to help their dad. The lower right quadrant represents either the near future or the recent past; the lower left represents the distant past; and either the far future or the death concept is shown in the upper left. For example, if someone drew on one sheet of paper several different places he was thinking of moving to, whatever place occupied the upper left would be the one he would move to.

A perfect example of the quadrant theory is illustrated by figure 21. A neighbor of mine stopped by and told me she was depressed, so I asked her to do a drawing for me. In the upper right (the present) she was walking downhill with four rays of sunshine behind her. "I am feeling down about my divorce and those are my four children. They are my sunshine," she said. In the lower right (near future or recent past) there were eight stick people in red (strong emotion), but she didn't know what they signified. The lower left (distant past) contained waves of seawater, and she said she'd grown up in a house on the beach. In the upper left quadrant (far future) she'd drawn black clouds. She believed these referred to her upcoming divorce.

Weeks later, after sending her kids out the door to catch the school bus, she took an overdose of sleeping pills to commit suicide. The amazing thing is that the children refused to get on the school bus when it arrived. Something told them they needed to go home, which they did, so they found their mother and saved her life. She awoke in the intensive care unit with eight angry members of her family standing around her bed (red stick people).

Susan Bach notes that movement and direction are also important in the drawings. A bus traveling down to the left side of the page would denote a downward spiral in the physical or emotional state, whereas one starting from the lower left and climbing up to the right can indicate improvement or climbing out from the darkest depths.[5]

One more caution must be mentioned here: the placement of objects in quadrants should be used only as a guide, for there are no rules cast in stone when dealing with individuals' subconscious language. Quadrant placement is not a science but a theory based on common traits seen in hundreds of people's drawings, so it may not always be applicable.

Numbers play a significant role and should be considered carefully, because they are one way that we store memories. Just as archetypes represent a larger idea, numbers can be meaningful, complex symbols. Jung said, "I have the distinct feeling that number is a key to the mystery, since it is just as much discovered as it is invented. It is quantity as well as meaning."[6] Numbers may appear in the drawing as numerical figures, such as the seven on the sail of a boat (fig. 65), or they can be quantities, like the number of green shrubs (fig. 24) or of windows on a plane (fig. 70).

Colors contain universal meanings: yellow represents energy; green is growth and life force; black symbolizes sadness or despair, and so on. Once again, however, caution must be advised, because people may have unique personal or cultural symbolic meanings. A color itself should never be judged as good or bad. In China, for example, red signifies good luck and prosperity, while in America it often represents the passion of anger or of love. The wise physician or therapist will ask his patient: "What does this color mean to you?" Interpretation of the drawing then becomes far more helpful to the patient and people involved in his care. Remember that the individual may actually have a gray house with a black roof (fig. 63), so we need to know the facts.

In general, black represents grief and despair. Red signifies strong emotions ranging from pain or anger to love and passion. Orange is symbolic of change, which can be a good thing if it is the color of your treatment. Yellow is energy, and you want to see it in your treatment, not your disease. Green, blue, and brown are all natural, life-supporting, healthy colors, but when they are pale, or especially when they fade in a series of pictures drawn over time, it can mean that the life force is fading. White signifies that something is being covered up, since the page is already white, just as pink or gray can represent red or black covered up emotionally. Purple symbolizes a healing property, spiritual growth, or a transformation, such as the transformation from being a living person to becoming spirit.

For further information, I heartily recommend two books I mentioned earlier, and whose authors have helped me in the past: *Life*

Paints Its Own Span by Susan Bach and *The Secret World of Drawings* by Gregg Furth.[7] Both books are entirely devoted to drawings.

Pictures can reveal problems that patients don't speak to their doctors about, often because the patients are unaware of them consciously. At the same time, their subconscious *is* aware, and art provides a visual language to get the problem across. I found it particularly helpful to show parents their children's drawings so they would see the messages their children were putting forth but not feel like I was criticizing them. When a boy portrayed himself like a black insect on the operating table (fig. 44), it revealed his lack of self-esteem. His parents could see he needed more than plastic surgery; he needed their love.

In family drawings it is important to pay close attention to facial expressions, bodies touching, and space between people. Missing people or missing body parts, people's positions, and any oddities or errors also reveal important areas of conflict. Freud pointed out that when a person's conscious mind is at variance with his subconscious, the conflict that the patient could not voice always escapes in the guise of an error or omission in his speaking, writing, or drawing. He believed there are no mistakes; that the subconscious is demanding attention.

When a nun with cancer handed me her drawing of her family members (fig. 68), their body positions revealed they were not open to each other. I told the nun she would have to let them know she needed their support or get help from someone else, because the family was simply not there to supply it.

You don't have to be sick to reap the benefits from creating drawings. You can use them to understand yourself and other people better and help them to know themselves better, too. With adults and seniors, comparison drawings of themselves today and themselves twenty-five years ago can be a revealing exercise that confirms their sense of self-acceptance and identity. Feelings of discontent will show up in the "today" picture when the self is depicted as fat, bald, and unhappy compared to twenty-five years ago, when the self was depicted as slim, happy, and with hair. This provides an opportunity to address the person's feelings in a beneficial way.

Among seniors, drawings often spark communication about who they were, who they are now, and who they can be. For example, one man drew only one picture and said, "That's me then and me now." He had never stopped giving love or caring for others; the nursing home he lived and died in now has a memorial to him in its library. When the younger generation who care for the residents of senior homes learn more about their clients through drawings such as these, they cease to see them as just a bunch of oldies; each resident becomes an individual, a human being with a story.

One example of using drawings for making important life decisions is beautifully illustrated by a medical student who came to me for advice. His dad, a doctor and a friend of mine, had died of cancer. The son had become unsure about whether he truly wanted to be a doctor, fearing that the pressure and emotions experienced by people in the profession were part of why his father got sick. I said to him, "Draw a picture of all the professions you're thinking that you might go into."

He came back and handed me three drawings. In the first (fig. 13), he was a politician. He was the only person in the picture who had an ear; he didn't have hands or feet, and neither did anybody else. There wasn't much color in the picture and it was framed in black, so I said "No, don't be a politician." When he handed me the next one (fig. 14), he said, "I could be a teacher." I advised him not to go for that either. All the nice colors were outside the window. Inside there were red desks, an emotional color, and nobody in the room had ears or feet, including him so I said he would feel trapped if he went into teaching. Then we looked at the last one (fig. 15), of him as a doctor. The one thing missing was the ear again, but I thought that related to his fears about his father, as if he were thinking: "What am I going to hear that's going to be a problem for me emotionally?" But the room was a healthy color with a green floor, plants growing, and a blue desk. He was reaching for the patient. The room had a door too. If things got tough, he could step out the door and take a vacation. His purple pants were a spiritual color. This showed that his connection to people was based on an awareness of life at physical, mental, and spiritual levels. He eventually became a psychiatrist, and he's happy at what he's doing.

DOCTOR'S R_{x}

Pick a situation, subject, problem, or decision you are considering. Draw your choices and observe the details the following day when you can view them intellectually — as if someone else did the drawing — and you are no longer consciously blind to the symbolism portrayed. Share the drawings with someone you trust. Ask that person to tell you what he or she sees in the picture and how it makes him or her feel. This person's comments, together with your own interpretation, will give you more insight into your problem and will help you to make a self-serving, authentic choice. Remember: you are the only one who knows the truth behind the symbolism, so don't let others impose their incorrect interpretation on your inner wisdom and knowingness.

Chapter 6

INTERPRETING THE DRAWINGS

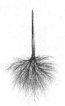

*I found that I could say things with colors and shapes that I couldn't
say in any other way — things that I had no words for.*

— GEORGIA O'KEEFFE

The following drawings are taken from my collection, which has been gathered over thirty years. The drawings were done by friends, family, colleagues, my patients, and patients under the care of other doctors. My commentary about them will help readers understand how each one was interpreted. In some cases, where appropriate and meaningful, I have mentioned the patient's outcome. The purpose of this commentary is not to relate personal histories but to introduce readers to the language of the subconscious through drawings, and to illustrate how each picture becomes a valuable resource, even when it is only a few lines scribbled on a page. Recent studies reveal how imagery can speed healing and reduce pain after surgery. The drawings reveal what images need to be created for this to happen in all aspects of life.

COLORS: WHAT THEY CAN REVEAL

FIGURE 1

The child artist has drawn a ball of color that is fairly well contained and controlled, but the colors are not in order, as they would be in a rainbow. The black section of the image suggests that something in the child's life is bothering her. The picture shows a lot of emotion (the reds) and all kinds of things going on in her life: purples = spiritual aspects; yellows = energy. But still, there is an issue that's buried, and it needs to be brought out and talked about. It's not a massive problem but something that's eating away deep within her. It looks as if her *life* is out of order, and not that she's experiencing a physical disorder. If the child had drawn herself and put some black in that image, then I would say it could represent a physical disease, but this more clearly signifies something emotional.

FIGURE 2

When the boy who drew this picture is happy and his life is in order, there is a rainbow; all his emotions are in order. But here the rainbow is between black clouds. When he's living in the rainbow, he feels good; so even when there's trouble in his life, he still maintains order and control of his feelings. The picture is filled in with blue and green — natural, healthy colors. His life is full, which is indicated by the fact that he took time to color the whole page. But still, there are things that limit his rainbow. I would ask him what problems he is experiencing — what's getting in the way and curtailing his happiness — and would work with him on any problem he then verbalized.

FIGURE 3

The colors on this balloon resemble a rainbow, but the colors have been rearranged so that red and orange are on the inside. This could mean the artist is burying or hiding the feelings they represent, rather than expressing them. The sun is present, but even it has red streaks in front of it. This implies he has an emotional issue he needs to deal with

— not a terrible one, because he's got a lot of healthy, natural colors here, and there's a blue cloud with yellow, not a black cloud. Helen Keller said if you face the sunshine, you'll never see the shadows, but it's hard for him to face the sunshine because, in his drawing, the cloud (his emotional issue) is getting in the way.

Because of the colors the artist has picked, I don't think the implied problem would be hard to resolve. I would ask him why the balloon is anchored, and why it's tied with three strings. Why isn't he in the balloon taking a nice trip? I would ask, "What's tying you down, what's limiting you and causing emotional tension?" The balloon also looks like a lightbulb, which could be his inner voice saying, "I need to bring light to the situation and resolve it." I would also ask him to count the little green plants and see if the number is meaningful to him.

FIGURE 4

Compare this drawing to the rainbow picture and notice how it makes you feel. It prompts you to ask, "What's going on in this kid's life?" It's messy, without order, and there's black in it. It could be the result of a parental or family problem, an illness, or any of a host of other things. The child needs help finding order in his or her life. The letters are purple, which indicates the artist is spiritual and not so sick he is going to become a spirit. All the feelings are there, out in the open, but they need to be expressed in a healthy way so that the problem can be resolved and the confusion cleared away.

FIGURE 5

This looks like coils of wire or yarn all tangled up. This is the central issue. It's so light and streaky; there's a lot of energy in it and total entanglement. Something has created that tangle and caused the problem. If black were not present, I'd say it's a matter of disorder, but the black here suggests a significant emotional issue that needs to be dealt with. The child needs to express her feelings and to get help untangling her life. Getting her straightened out will take a lot more work than helping the child who drew figure 4.

ANATOMY: INNER KNOWLEDGE
OF STRUCTURES AND DISEASE

FIGURE 6

Following an appendectomy, a young boy's abdomen was distended, meaning he was filling with gas because his intestine hadn't started working again. My immediate worry was whether there was an obstruction, which would require another surgery to relieve it. I asked him to draw a picture of himself. He drew an x-ray on the wall, although there was no x-ray-viewing screen in his room, so I paid close attention to the x-ray. In the x-ray, the big white area is his stomach, and the coils represent his intestine. When you have intestinal obstruction, the small intestine fills with gas and fluid because it can't empty out, but here it is neatly folded, with no distention. In addition, the boy chose brown and blue, healthy colors, rather than red and black, which would have suggested there was a problem.

These details led me to believe his intestines must simply be recovering from the original infection and the anesthetic drugs, and that he had no intestinal obstruction. Having learned through experience to trust patients' drawings, I continued to observe him and treat him symptomatically. In a few days his intestines were working again, and he began to pass gas. His body had just needed more time than usual to recover, and no further surgery was required.

FIGURE 7

A male patient with some symptoms of appendicitis drew this picture and threw it in the wastebasket. I pulled it out and studied the picture. An appendix looks like one finger of a glove attached to the intestine, much like the arms and legs in this picture. When it becomes obstructed by feces or something else, it becomes engorged and inflamed. Observe the little ball at the end of this figure's arm. It looks like a blockage; also note the swollen extremities, lacking hands or feet, and the empty spaces. The color is orange, which refers to change; after an operation, the patient would be different. This drawing, coupled with his symptoms, led me to believe he did have appendicitis and that he needed surgery. We operated and confirmed the diagnosis.

FIGURES 8 AND 9

When this boy was wheeled into the operating room, he gave me two drawings, even though I hadn't asked him to draw anything. Handing me figure 8, he said, "This is like before the operation," and handing me figure 9, he said, "And this is like after the operation." Stop and look. This is a good example of how the subconscious uses visual language. What operation do you think he had? The boy drew airplanes, but you can see what part of the anatomy they represented. Another word that refers to a penis is cock; and here the pilot is, sitting in a cockpit. In figure 8, the foreskin is covering the penis, and in figure 9 the foreskin is gone and the penis is exposed.

In the first drawing, the cockpit is open and the pilot's head is sticking out, but in the after-surgery image the artist closes the cockpit and is hiding the pilot inside. It says to me that he's going to protect his penis for the rest of his life and not let anything like this happen to it again. It's interesting that the bullets from the gun mounted on the wing change from droplets, in the first picture, to straight lines in the second. I'd say the straight lines look more powerful, more forceful. He knows it will be ready to go to work and do what it needs to do. And blue is a healthy color. So he's not feeling pain or distress at the prospect of surgery. This drawing says the circumcision is an okay thing for him.

FIGURES 10 AND 11

These two images were drawn by brothers. Timothy drew his house (fig. 10), and it looks like a phallic symbol in red, a sign of emotion, which relates to his surgery (circumcision). And he put fourteen apples on his tree, which may relate to people in the family, a date, or some other quantity. He used healthy colors for the sun (yellow = energy), tree (green = life), and swing set (blue = health). The swings are a source of fun, with the red representing him, and the blue, his brother. The mailbox flag is up and, along with its color (brown = nourishing earth), its existence suggests he has no trouble communicating his feelings; the chimney on the house gives him an outlet to relieve pressure and worry. This picture suggests he will be okay.

Thomas, too, drew a phallic house (fig. 11), in purple with nine windows on one side of the house and one window at the end of the attic. His tree had nine apples close together and one positioned at the edge of the tree. Nine and one are significant because he repeats the pattern, and had he been my patient I would have asked him whether those numbers held any meaning. His colors are healthy, but the frame he added to the edges of the paper suggests he feels limited or restricted; and he has no chimney to release pressure and worry.

FIGURE 12

Look at these sails. It's easy to see this woman has breast cancer. The birds are the people in her life who have difficulty coping with her cancer, and so they are black. The sun has seven rays but is partly out of the picture. The boat represents her and the current problem, and it is outlined in black and red (grief, pain, worry) and is sailing on rough seas. Nobody is in the boat; it appears to be tossed about, with only the wind controlling the sails, which reveals what she is experiencing.

THE FUTURE, DEATH, AND INTUITION: CONSCIOUS OR UNCONSCIOUS KNOWING

FIGURES 13, 14, AND 15

In the previous chapter I referred to the medical student who came to me seeking advice about his career choice after his father, a doctor, died from cancer. The student was worried that the physical and emotional demands of being a doctor had contributed to his father's disease. I told him to draw himself in the occupations he was considering. In figure 13, he's a politician. In figure 14, he is a teacher. Neither of these looked promising. His drawing of the doctor (fig. 15) was the most pleasant scene, with its healthy colors, images, and actions. I recommended that he stay in medical school and he did. He became a psychiatrist, which turned out to be the right profession for him.

FIGURES 16 AND 17

I asked medical students to draw pictures of themselves working as doctors, and figures 16 and 17 represent two extremes from that class. Almost all the students, whether male or female, drew the doctor sitting behind a desk with a diploma on the wall, but they depicted no patients or other people in the same room. Figure 16 blew my mind. There's a vague face on the lower right, but it's unclear whether it represents the doctor or the patient. It appears as if it may signify an intellect, not a human being, because only the head is present. And what else does this doctor have? Books, a computer, a name, vegetables, pills — it's not about people. This drawing is not about caring for people but about treating disease. The individual who drew it would label patients: "You have a migraine headache, or you have cancer; here take this." Or: "If you're depressed, take that." I can't imagine this artist functioning as a doctor unless she were to go into research, working only in the laboratory instead of with patients.

At the other extreme is a wonderful picture from the same class (fig. 17). *This* is what being a doctor is all about. The artist depicts himself kneeling down, so he's at the patient's level. Look at that arm — he's become one with her. He's making eye contact, smiling, and giving her a tissue. His body is saying there's hope. He has a stethoscope, but it's not what he uses to touch the patient. If students depict themselves touching a patient, usually they show themselves doing so with the stethoscope or some other instrument, not their hands.

Among patients' drawings, the most encouraging ones show people in their room — the operating room, or their hospital room where they are supposed to be in isolation receiving a bone marrow transplant — and the doctor is with them, touching them. When patients envision their doctors without a cap, mask, and gown on, which they would wear in the sterile environment of a real operating room, the symbolism is beautiful. It suggests a personal relationship and a positive outcome.

FIGURE 18

The man who drew this was afraid to have chemotherapy and refused treatment. But the yellow energy flowing to his cancer revealed that his intuition knew it would be good for him. Intellect and intuition don't always agree. Whether you decide to have a treatment or not, you don't want to be in conflict about it. After understanding what his inner voice was saying, he decided to go ahead, and it proved to be the right decision.

FIGURES 19 AND 20

These two images were drawn by a doctor who had developed cancer. In figure 19, the three birds are his children. The drooping wings mean they're having emotional problems dealing with their father's illness. The fish (a spiritual symbol) is out of the water and facing west, where the sun sets, revealing how he feels about what he is facing. He's also sailing away from the sun and his kids. He and his wife are in the boat, on this journey together, and they're orange (which signals an upcoming change). I hope the yellow sail and purple boat are about the couple's faith, spiritual growth, and transformation — not a sign that he is planning to die. He's sitting, and the lines depicting the boat's outline are under his feet, so he's not tied down; he's able to get out. But the lines go over his wife, holding her body down. He's got the sail and the tiller, so even though she's with him on the journey, he isn't letting her help him. This is not survival behavior. It's as if he's trying to protect the family by not telling them how he feels (one hand is behind his back). He's got all the controls, and when he doesn't let them help him, they feel worse.

After a little therapy, the doctor drew figure 20. Notice the bright colors of his kids (the birds) and how their wings go up. He's now sailing toward the sun (the far future), and rays of energy are emanating from it. Count the rays; he's got a good number of years ahead of him. The fish has turned around and looks more powerful, with better color. It is facing the east, where the sun rises — and when you face the sun, you see no shadows. The four waves represent completeness. The wind is in his sail; he doesn't have to hold or control it, and he and his wife are holding hands. They're smiling; they're on the journey together and no longer separated. They have eyes and noses. God breathed life into Adam through his nostrils. If you don't have a nose, how do you breathe life? He's got an ear, so his wife can talk to him, and he's listening to her.

FIGURE 21

The woman who drew this was consciously unaware not only that her drawing would predict her suicide attempt but also that her children, symbolized by four rays of sunshine, would save her, and that eight members of her family would be there when she woke up in the hospital. I folded the drawing into quadrants to show how present, past, and future were all represented.

FIGURES 22 AND 23

The color orange means change, and when seven-year-old Monica wrote her name in black on orange (fig. 22), it signaled that she was not happy about having surgery. In the room where Monica was going to have her surgery, two yellow lights, which you could reach up to adjust and focus on the operation, hung over the operating table (fig. 23). The lights were attached to bendable arms, which could be maneuvered to direct the light, and at the elbow a black knob would tighten to hold the light in place. What is really interesting here is that Monica had never been in the operating room. Even so, she drew a room like a box, and at both ends are two yellow lights with two black knobs on each of them. During an operation, the patient lies on a white sheet, and is then covered with a sterile blue sheet that has an opening positioned over the surgical area. Here Monica has drawn the white and blue sheets, and she is the pink figure in the center. She also drew four lines above her head. In the operating room, there is a scrub nurse, an anesthesiologist, and myself, as well as a circulating nurse — someone who isn't scrubbed in and who can leave the room and get whatever equipment the surgeon may need. In the drawing, the circulating nurse is represented by a line that partly crosses the room's border. Monica intuitively knew that this is a person who can come and go and who wouldn't remain in the room with her the whole time.

This picture is what changed people's thinking at the hospital. Many of them had thought I was nuts to glean information from drawings, but this was a child who drew key elements of the operating room despite having never seen it. So where did this picture come from? After Monica's drawing impressed people at the hospital, they were converted, and my patients' drawings became a lot more interesting than x-rays and scans.

FIGURE 24

The green shrubs in this woman's drawing turned out to be a prediction of how long she would live: she was buried nearly three years to the day after she drew it.

FIGURES 25 AND 26

Before our daughter got married, I said to her and her fiancé, "Why don't you each draw two pictures — one of yourself and one of the two of you as a couple?" Our daughter drew on the front and back of one piece of paper, which is meaningful because you can hold it up to the light and the self-portrait becomes superimposed on the couple on the opposite side. (If the person or family members are positioned so they're standing on you, your family is a problem.) When I held this up to the light, her raised hand was on his head and her other hand was on her heart. I said, "If he's in his head and you are in your heart, you're going to have a problem."

The drawing of the couple (fig. 25) shows her pulling him to get him to walk in her direction, but he isn't even looking at her. They do have ears, but hers are black because what she hears from him is causing her to despair. In her self-portrait (fig. 26) she is wearing orange shoes, yet with him she is wearing black ones. She's got bigger fingers in the self-portrait, so she's got a better grip on things when she's not with him. I said, "Between his head and your heart, you've got to find a way to communicate with each other and work things out if your relationship is going to survive." But they never did. One of their sons was born with a serious genetic metabolic problem; and when that was added to the situation, divorce was the ultimate outcome.

FIGURE 27

This was drawn by a doctor who had cancer and whose kids were grown. He wondered how his kids were doing. I said, "Draw a picture of your family for me." He said, "They're all over the country; what's that going to tell me?" I told him he'd intuitively know what was going on, and so he brought in this picture. The first thing I told him was to stop labeling his kids. He's written beneath them: "Yale," "Architect," "Attorney," and so on, and everybody's professional. So I asked him, "If you had a drug addict, a school dropout, and a mass murderer, would you write those details in?" He laughed and shook his head. "Don't label your kids," I told him.

As I looked over the drawing, it was fairly obvious which of his children he needed to talk to. I always say that being an attorney is a serious illness. One attorney told me, "While learning to think, I almost forgot how to feel." And that's what had happened to this doctor's attorney child: he's all in black, he isn't touching anybody in the family, and I'm sure from this picture he had been living totally in his head. He needed contact with his family, and he needed encouragement to express his feelings. His dad was able to get in touch with him and help him work that out.

NATURE: A MIRROR OF OUR INTERNAL ENVIRONMENT

FIGURE 28

We perceive trees as symbols for human beings: for our families, our lives, and our bodies. When you draw a tree, usually the part of the tree beneath the ground — the roots — symbolizes your unconscious. It can also refer to your family's roots. The tree's trunk represents your body and what's going on in your life; the top branches of the tree can represent the future and your growth and consciousness.

The tree in figure 28 is not centered over the roots; the artist may be disconnected from her family. The hole in the trunk suggests that something is eating a hole in her or in her life. I don't think the creature depicted inside the hole represents a disease, but a person who is eating her up. Look at the confusion of the branches. There's life, but where is it going? It's a tangled mess. This artist needs to resolve a relationship with her family, so I would ask, "Who's eating a hole in you?" It is possible that the object inside the trunk could be the patient herself — represented by a child in the womb of the tree. She needs to create her own authentic life and not live the life imposed on her by others. She needs to be born again as her true self.

FIGURE 29

This picture shows what we're all here to do. Life is meant to be an opportunity for us to grow and blossom in a healthy way. This is such a beautiful picture, with the yellow energy in the background, the sunlight bathing the flower, and the healthy green, a sign of life. When children have cancer and are not doing well, the colors fade and become very light. But this picture shows a person who is blossoming, reaching up and out to all that is good in life.

FIGURE 30

When peoples' arms are up, this can represent many different emotions. But look at this tree: it has thin, tangled branches, all drawn in emotional colors. The two figures are standing on the ground, so they do have some support beneath them; often people draw themselves floating in the air, with no support. The feet of these two point in opposite directions, indicating they really need to make up their minds, decide where they are going. It's also hard to see anything that looks like a trunk on this tree; there's only one very thin line. Their life together needs to be strengthened, brought into order. Neither person has been drawn with a nose, showing that their lives are uninspiring — they need to make a more vibrant life for themselves and not live on an island.

FIGURE 31

Birds almost always represent the people in your life. In this drawing, three birds are together in front of the moon and one is on its own. Birds in black may represent people who are causing you grief and despair or experiencing it themselves. The night sky has some color along with the black, but it is not a pleasant-looking sky. The ship is drawn in two emotional colors, black for grief or despair, and red, the emotional color, which could be love but in most cases represents pain or conflict. When the patient's life journey (the boat) is black and red, I don't get a very good feeling about his state. Also, who's sailing it? Which way is it going? One of the lines goes over the sail, making it look stuck — almost as if in a whirlpool — and it's tied to the horizon line. The purple water could signify some kind of spiritual journey, but the ship needs help, in the sense that it needs somebody to guide it and deal with the painful emotions of the journey this person is on. The little birds may be people in the artist's life, but they don't look as if they're going to be very helpful. So this person must ask for help. When you need help, ask for it; that's survival behavior.

FIGURE 32

The snow on the three mountains wasn't drawn with white crayon, but still, snow is covering something, so I would ask the artist: Are three people, or three things in your life, getting in your way, and are you covering up your feelings about it? The sun is in the future quadrant, which gives a feeling of hope, but there are no rays (joy) coming down into the picture. The path travels from the recent past (the lower right) into the far future (the upper left) and becomes a little skinny, which will make it hard to stay on that path.

Just as there are three mountains, there are three big trees. One of these trees is alive; the other two look dead or dormant. If they represent people, then no one is nourishing them, and they, like that pathway, are beginning to die out. It's as if their life force is fading. Even the fir trees have black trunks, which could symbolize their problems. Purple mountains are spiritual symbols, and a Christmas-type tree can be spiritual, too, but something has drained the life out of the two deciduous trees, which may represent a parent and child. I'd also ask the artist: Does the number five mean anything to you? The fence, with its five posts, stands in the quadrant of the picture that represents the past. At the base of each post stands some healthy green growth. There are also a few more trees standing in the past. But since all the evergreen trees are black at the base, even though they appear healthy otherwise, there's conflict. I think something in the artist's past that needs to grow is being held back by this fence, and the artist needs therapy to bring it out.

FIGURE 33

This drawing is another kind of rainbow, with red, yellow, orange, purple, and green, and it's full of life. Even though the colors are not in rainbow order, the drawing has order — a balance — and it's beautiful. The pitcher rests on a brown stand, a strong, earthy color, so it's got support; the handle suggests you can get a grip on it, pick it up, and take it with you. You can fill this pitcher with water to sustain the flowers. This drawing gives me a good feeling about the person's life. I would ask the artist: "Why are there four yellow flowers, two purples, and so on?" or "Why are there eight flowers?" If the number eight doesn't apply to anything specific to the artist, it can mean that there is a new beginning, or that one is coming soon.

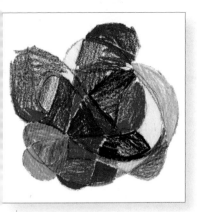

figure 1 (see page 74)

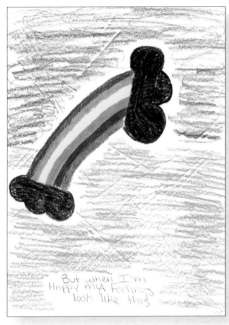

figure 2 (see page 74)

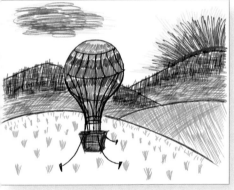

figure 3 (see pages 74–75)

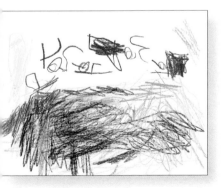

figure 4 (see page 75)

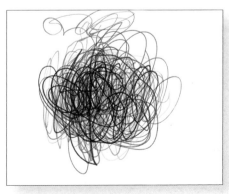

figure 5 (see page 75)

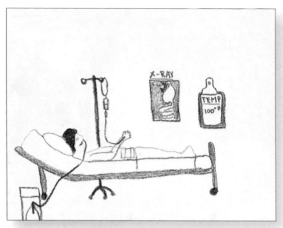

figure 6 (see page 76)

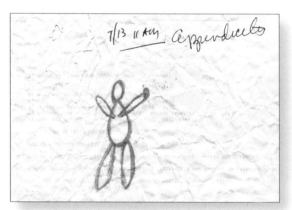

figure 7 (see pages 76–77)

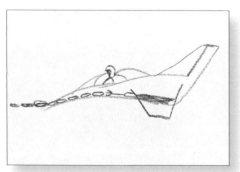

figure 8 (see page 77)

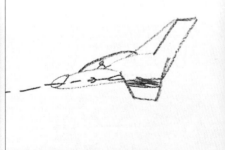

figure 9 (see page 77)

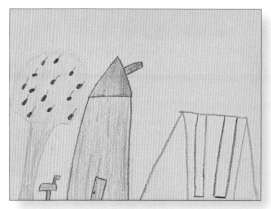

figure 10 (see pages 77–78)

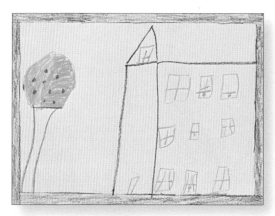

figure 11 (see pages 77–78)

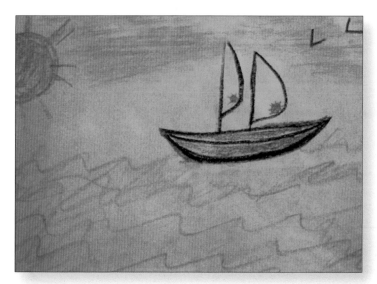

figure 12 (see pages 67, 78)

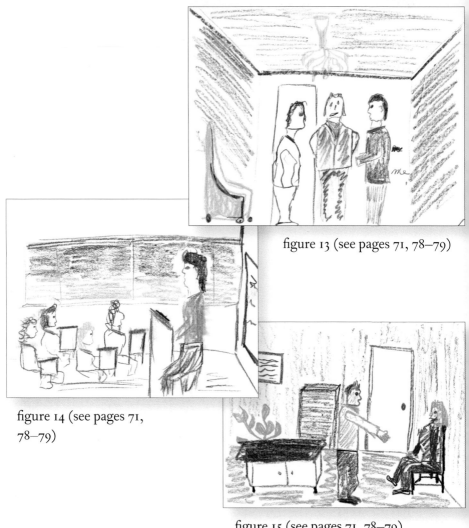

figure 13 (see pages 71, 78–79)

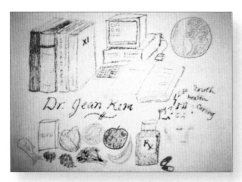

figure 14 (see pages 71, 78–79)

figure 15 (see pages 71, 78–79)

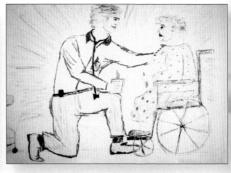

figure 16 (see pages 79–80)

figure 17 (see pages 79–80)

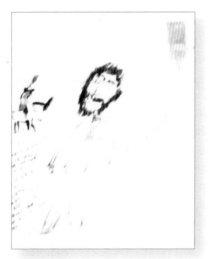

figure 18 (see pages 58, 80)

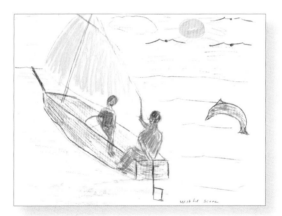

figure 19 (see pages 67, 80–81)

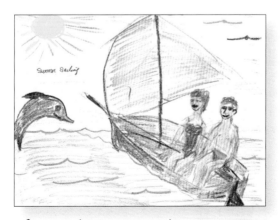

figure 20 (see pages 80–81)

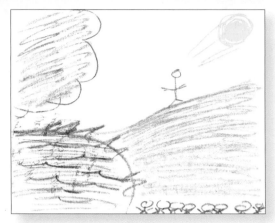

figure 21 (see pages 68, 81)

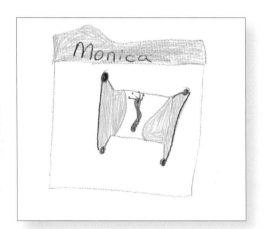

figure 22 (see pages 43, 81–82)

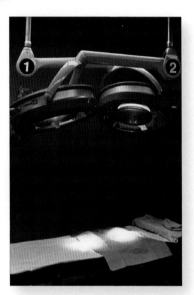

figure 23 (see pages 81–82)

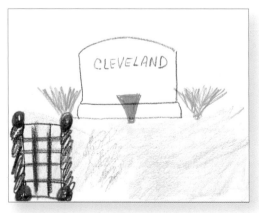

figure 24 (see pages 67, 69, 82)

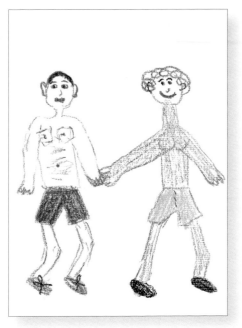

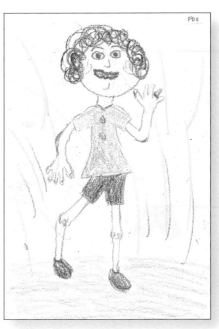

figure 25 (see pages 82–83)

figure 26 (see pages 82–83)

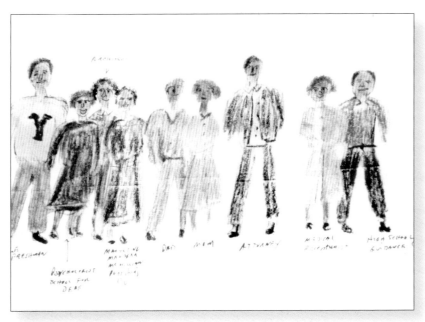

figure 27 (see page 83)

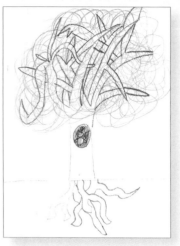

figure 28 (see page 84)

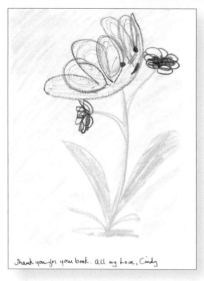

Thank you for your book. all my love, Cindy

figure 29 (see page 84)

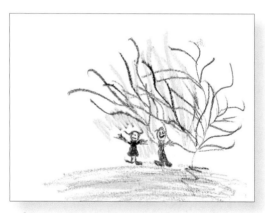

figure 30 (see pages 84–85)

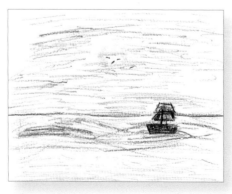

figure 31 (see page 85)

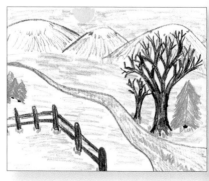

figure 32 (see pages 85–86)

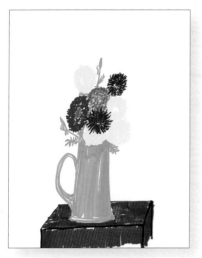

figure 33 (see page 86)

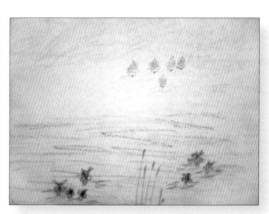

figure 34 (see page 87)

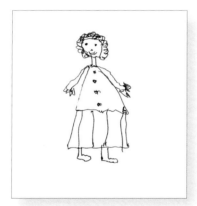

figure 35 (see pages 87–88)

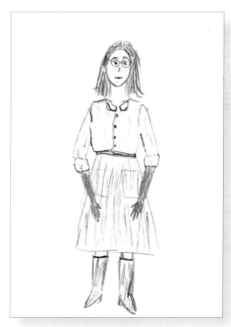

figure 36 (see page 88)

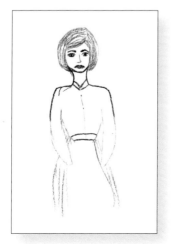

figure 37 (see pages 88–89)

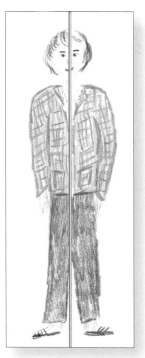

figure 38 (see pages 89–90)

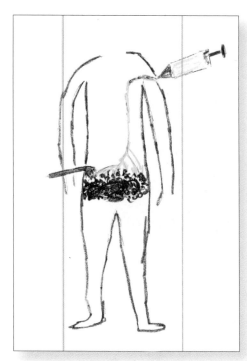

figure 39 (see pages 89–90)

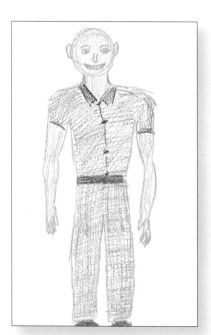

figure 40 (see page 90)

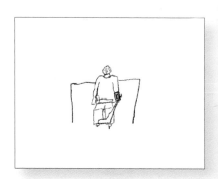

figure 41 (see pages 90–91)

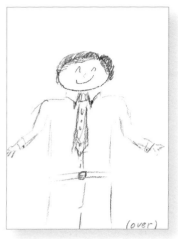

figure 42 (see page 91)

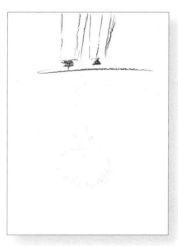

figure 43 (see page 91)

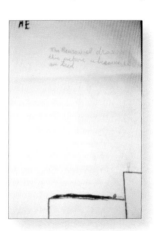

figure 44 (see pages 70, 91–92)

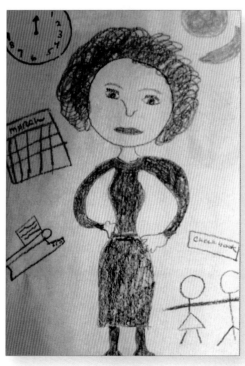

figure 45 (see pages 62, 92)

figure 46 (see pages 92–93)

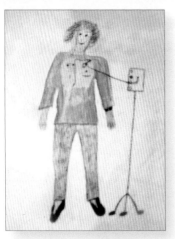

figure 47 (see pages 93, 129)

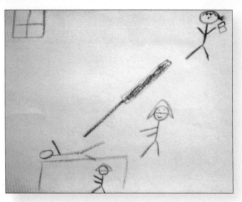

figure 48 (see page 94)

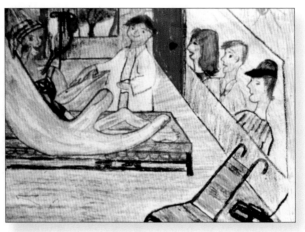

figure 49 (see pages 94–95)

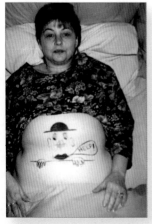

figure 50 (see page 95)

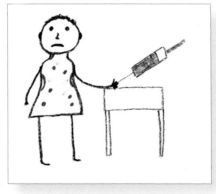

figure 51 (see pages 95–96)

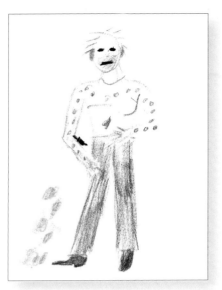

figure 52 (see pages 60, 96–97)

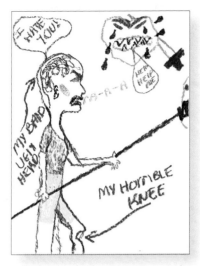

figure 53 (see page 97)

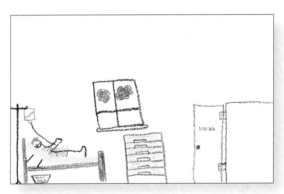

figure 54 (see pages 98–99)

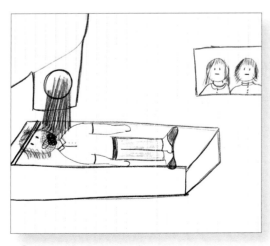

figure 55 (see page 99)

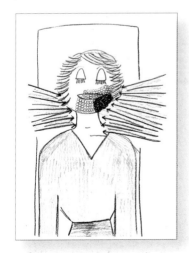

figure 56 (see page 99)

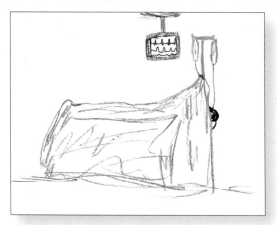

figure 57 (see pages 59, 99–100)

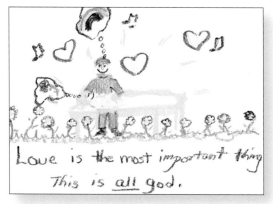

figure 58 (see pages 60, 100)

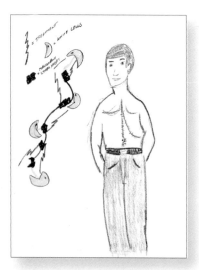

figure 59 (see pages 60, 100–101)

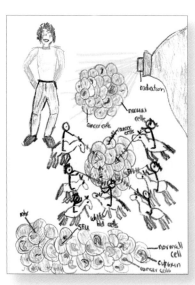

figure 60 (see page 101)

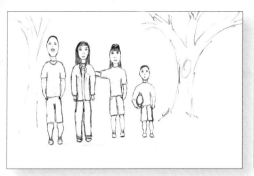

figure 61 (see pages 62, 101)

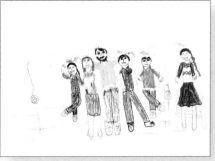

figure 62 (see pages 64, 102)

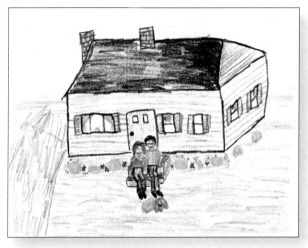

figure 63 (see pages 69, 102)

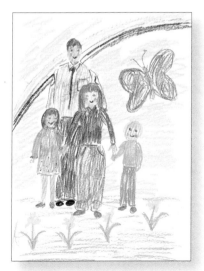

figure 64 (see pages 60, 102–3)

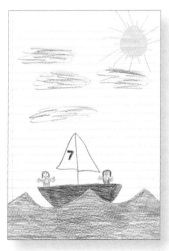

figure 65 (see pages 69, 103)

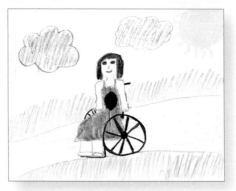

figure 66 (see pages 103–4)

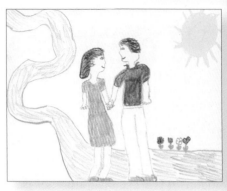

figure 67 (see pages 103–4)

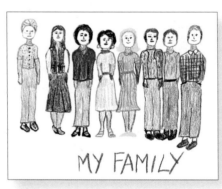

figure 68 (see pages 70, 104–5)

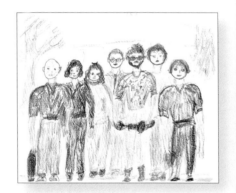

figure 69 (see pages 105–6)

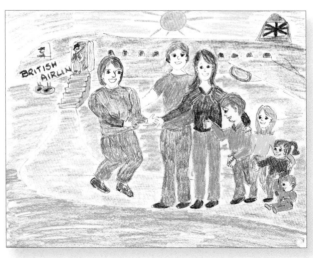

figure 70 (see pages 69, 106, 205)

Figure 34

My wife, Bobbie, drew this outdoor scene with five trees at the top of the page. We have five children, and at the time she drew this, one of our kids was causing us a problem. He was the one who stands out of line. I was trying to get him to go off to college and not simply hang around the house complaining all the time. He's a bright kid with a lot of energy, but he found school boring. When he was younger, and my wife and I were away on vacation, he would hide in the closet and read books all day instead of going to school. So I was trying to get him to go out and study something of interest.

When Bobbie drew this, two of our children were away and three were at home. But look at the bottom of the picture, where there are seven flowers (representing all of us). On the bottom left are the twins, my wife, and me. The third flower has gone to the other side of the cattails, so this told me he was going to leave home, which eliminated the pressure completely. There were six cattails. Six weeks from the day of this drawing, our son got in his car, drove to Denver, and joined his brother at school there. This picture still impresses me, and we keep it hanging in our house.

SELF-IMAGE: SEEING HOW SELF-WORTH AFFECTS OUR BODIES

Figure 35

This young woman was admitted to the hospital because she was literally starving herself to death. Everybody there was angry at her and demanded to know why she was doing this. And they were treating her rudely. So I went in and said, "Honey, draw me a picture," and she drew this. I took it out to everybody and told them, "Look, this is a picture of herself. Do you understand the problem she is dealing with now? Her image of herself is that of a pregnant-looking, obese woman." When they realized how she saw herself, they all calmed down and began treating her differently.

What I like about the drawing is that both feet are headed toward the east. I knew that, with therapy, she was heading in the right direction, and that because they weren't pointing opposite ways, she was not confused or conflicted. She needed bigger fingers, so she could get a grip on things. The four buttons may have meant something to her. She was beginning to find herself, symbolized by her sticking her neck out a little. Having only dots for a nose suggests she needed to find something that would inspire her, and if she did, she would develop into a whole person, which would be shown by the use of color rather than black lines. Without self-love, you cannot see your true self in the mirror and accept yourself as worth loving; you see only what's wrong.

FIGURE 36

What is interesting about this girl's picture is her arms: she's got hands, but they are tied down where the line of her dress goes over the arms. She's got all the parts, including eyes, nose, and mouth, and she fills the page, which says something positive about her self-esteem when compared to the small self-portrait drawn by the anorexic woman. But I want to ask her, "What has tied you down? What do you need to reach out for?" Her arms are brown and her face is white; it could be that coloring her arms dark reveals her difficulty in reaching out and doing what she needs to do. She's a white person with brown arms. It's as if she's afraid of being judged. Her feet are not pointed in the same direction, indicating a little indecision. Perhaps she's been criticized by others, who have told her, "You shouldn't do that."

FIGURE 37

You give somebody a box of crayons, and look what she does with it. Except for the red eyes and mouth, the figure is drawn in all black. She has eyes, a nose, and a mouth, but no ears, hands, or feet. This speaks of her depression. At least she didn't draw a smile on her face and deny her feelings — most people who are totally depressed still show themselves with a big grin. Also, the line is darker over the shoulders, so she's carrying a burden. I would ask her, "What is going on?" She has depicted herself as having nothing to remedy the situation with; she's feeling helpless. She needs help with learning how to reach out; how to grow some feet, move around, and do what needs to be done. Her belt is almost too tight, as if signaling that something in her life is constricting her. She has to learn to listen to her feelings the same way we respond to hunger and seek the nourishment we need.

FIGURES 38 AND 39

Figure 38 was drawn on the folded-in sides of a sheet of paper, so that the person you see here opens up like a book. The colors of the outer image are healthy and have energy, but the person's hands are mostly tucked in (the artist can't "handle" what she's facing), and the feet are turned in opposite directions (she's indecisive). The shoulders are wide, as if she is carrying a burden by herself. The image fills the page, so her self-esteem is good. When I asked the artist why she had folded the page, she opened it. Now see what's inside: In figure 39, her body is depersonalized. The artist is shown getting chemotherapy, which is yellow (representing energy), and it's going straight to the tumor, a good thing (fewer side effects). But look at her — she doesn't have a head, doesn't have hands, her feet are aimed in opposite directions, and her body is red, so I'd say she's feeling totally helpless and doesn't know what to do. Somebody else prescribed the treatment, and she thinks she *has* to go through with it.

Her treatment should be the result of her own decision and not about the doctor prescribing it. Yet she has hidden her misgivings under the folded page. I recommended that the patient either quit the treatment or change her attitude toward it. If you're going through hell, speak up; don't hide it from people. Take care of yourself and ask others to support you. What she needed to do was to empower herself and do the treatment only because it was her choice, not someone else's. That way she would have far fewer problems. Ten times a day for three or four minutes, she should visualize herself getting treatment, having a beautiful result with no side effects, and going home rejuvenated and healthy. When you feel helpless, or feel as if you're being poisoned by your treatment, you create the worst possible result.

I was watching something on public TV in which a psychologist discussed a research project that involved volunteers undergoing a functional brain scan that registers brain activity as it happens. In each trial they would hold up a hand in front of the person and watch which parts of the brain registered activity on the monitor. When the hand was taken away, the activity stopped in those areas. The psychologist noted that if you took the hand away and said to the person, "Close your eyes and imagine a hand," the brain on the imaging screen would light up in the same areas as before, showing the same activity, just as if the person were looking at an actual hand. So when you picture yourself getting treatment and doing well, it's as if you are. It makes an enormous difference.

FIGURE 40

That's me. Look at how big the shoulders are. I'm taking on too much, if you know what I mean. But I filled the page, which means my self-esteem is good; the colors are natural colors. I've got all the necessary parts — nose, mouth, eyes, and ears. It's a genuine smile, not a deceptive one. I've got four buttons on my shirt— to me that might be a number symbolizing completeness. My feet are on the ground. Even when you know what you're drawing, it's amazing how little details sneak in. If you look like you've got more muscles than in reality, you're trying to be the strong one and are not giving yourself the same good care that you give other people. I shouldn't do so much; I need to take care of myself and take it easy. Then if I drew another picture, it might be a little less muscular but healthier.

FIGURE 41

In contrast to the previous drawing, consider this image drawn by our neighbor's son, who was depressed. The boy's body doesn't fill the picture; he's a speck on the page, and he's depicted himself all in black, the goalie on a hockey team. What does he have to face? A goalie has to put up with everybody shooting hard black objects at him. The symbolism contained in that image is so clear, with the blackness of depression, the small self-image — and the way he holds his stick suggests he's expecting more troubles to come at him. This kid really needed help.

FIGURES 42 AND 43

This boy came into my office and drew a picture of himself that filled the page. Because of the purple, I could see that he's a spiritual guy, but in his picture he has no legs (fig. 42). I didn't notice that he'd written the word *over* on it. So I said, "What's the matter? You don't have legs. Are you feeling stuck or trapped?" And he said, "Turn the page over." On the other side of the paper, there he is with support under his feet (fig. 43). I fill one page when I draw myself, but this guy needs two pages. There's no need to worry about his self-esteem. If he takes two pages and has support, he'll make it. This drawing tells me he's doing okay.

FIGURE 44

This boy said, "Doctor Siegel, the kids are teasing me in the locker room at my school, and I want you to circumcise me so they stop making fun of me." I told him, "Draw a picture of yourself in the operating room," and handed him a whole box of crayons, with black, white, brown, and every color of the rainbow. What did he do but pull out a black crayon, write "Me" in black, and draw a black insect on the operating table. Then he wrote above it: "The reason I drew this picture is because I'm tired." I knew that wasn't why he drew this picture; it was how he felt about himself. If he had felt he was a beautiful child and was loved, he could have drawn himself as a beautiful young man who did or did not want a circumcision. I said, "Okay, you don't want kids to tease you? We can go ahead with the circumcision." But I showed the picture to his parents and told them, "I'll go ahead with the circumcision to help him, but he can spend his life seeing plastic surgeons and never feel beautiful when he looks in the mirror. What he needs most is your love."

I saw the same thing among personal health trainers at a convention. I asked them, "What should I hang up in the lobby of every public building to convey the message: 'Look at how beautiful and meaningful life is'?" They yelled out things like: "Butterflies!" "Rainbows!" "Baby pictures!" — until I said, "No, you hang up a mirror." When the first thought in your mind is a mirror, it signifies total acceptance and love of self. When we accept ourselves as God's creation, seeing beauty and meaning in what we are, just as we are, we accept others as God's creation too. Children find self-worth initially through their parents' love and acceptance; once they have that, they don't have to worry about how they look — about what their friends say and what the neighbors think. If they experience indifference and rejection from their parents, it can be disastrous.

FIGURE 45

This drawing was done by a reporter who interviewed me. When she drew a clock with only one hand, pointing to twelve, I realized her unconscious was demanding that she pay attention to a past traumatic experience, one that she needed therapeutic help to heal.

FIGURE 46

I show this picture at lectures and ask people, "Who do you think would produce detailed *written instructions* on how to draw a picture, when all I have asked the person to do is draw a picture?" When I say, "It was a male engineer," everybody laughs. He wrote at the top: "I have difficulty drawing." What's he worried about? It wasn't an art class; he wasn't getting graded. He didn't simply add a few words to label things, as some people do, but wrote a whole page of instructions. He was trying to control everything in his life by using his head. What is interesting is that this event still made an enormous difference to him, because I told him, "You're living in your head, not your feelings. The engineer part of you is having trouble with relationships; and just as lawyers do, you're thinking and measuring, not using your heart." That really struck him.

About fifteen years later, I showed this slide during a lecture at Yale, and afterward a man from the audience came to me and said, "That's my father's handwriting. When you told him he was relying entirely on his intellect, and not feeling his emotions, it changed him. It made such a difference for him and helped him survive his cancer." So I made a print of it and gave it to the son.

Some people are so afraid of drawing that they'll get their kid to do the drawing for them. I'll say to them, "You're fighting cancer and you're afraid to do a drawing?" One ten-year-old boy drew his mother's picture for her, giving it a big head and a fake smile. So he understood — she was living in her head, out of touch with her feelings.

TREATMENT: HOW WE PERCEIVE
AFFECTS HOW WE EXPERIENCE

FIGURE 47

This artist had a sense of humor that helped her survive. Here she has drawn herself getting chemotherapy, and she shows it flowing to all parts of her body — so she's unconsciously setting herself up to have plenty of side effects. She's attached to the pump that delivers the intravenous therapy over the course of an entire day and evening, one of several sessions that would happen over a period of months. She told me, "I'm tired of dragging this thing around." She really was ready to quit and die. So I looked at her and said, "You know, you're the Draggin' Lady" — a play on the name *Dragon Lady* — and she burst out laughing. Dragons became her symbols for her white blood cells during visualization sessions, and she did remarkably well from that moment on. She had no trouble with the treatment or anything else, because she became the Dragon Lady.

Doctors could benefit from learning psychological techniques for dealing with people, such as the play on words I used to entertain and energize the "Dragon Lady." I also use a technique I call Paradox, in which I do the opposite of what a patient may expect me to do. For example, when somebody comes in and says, "They told me I have a week to live," I say, "It looks to me like a couple of days." The patient will look at me, shocked, and then get it; I'm only teasing. What I've said is so outrageous that the patient bursts out laughing. Then we begin to talk, and the tension is gone. Using Paradox helps to shift the patient's thinking to something more positive, which in turn affects their experience of treatment. The resulting outcome will be more life enhancing, so I frequently deceive people into health.

The following drawings show two patients' different emotional responses to their treatments. These clearly illustrate why positive attitudes can play an important role in healing.

FIGURE 48

Here's somebody getting a bone marrow transplant, and it looks like it's happening in a prison. The window admits no sunshine, and there's nothing nice outside. The nurses are stick figures with no hands, and they aren't touching the patient. The patient has only one arm and no eyes, ears, or nose, and so no way to express herself. She's simply lying on a table as an enormous needle comes at her. This looks like a nightmare, not a healing therapy. A person who does a drawing like this needs to go home and visualize the treatment in a different way, as something therapeutic, until she can see it working to her benefit. I have a CD called *Getting Ready* that helps people "reprogram" themselves by means of guided visualization. I would have recommended it to this patient, because it would have entirely altered her response to and the outcome of her treatment. Now, let's compare it to the next picture, figure 49.

FIGURE 49

This is the scene of a bone marrow transplant, and that's God's hand supporting the patient. The IV is running; the doctor is in the room.

The doctor would normally have a cap, mask, and gown on, yet in this picture he doesn't, and he's touching her, not with a stethoscope, but with his hand — as a human being — and he's smiling. Although the picture has faded with age, you can still see the rainbow of life in the room with her, symbolized by the colors on the chair. It looks as if she's on a cruise vacation, not having a difficult procedure in hospital. There's light shining down on her; the door is red, an emotional color, which indicates that it's her doorway back to life. In one window stands the tree of life, a healthy-looking tree. Her family is waiting for her at the other window. She's got the CD player for her visualization therapy and everything in the room that she needs. I don't worry about a patient like this. Studies reveal that people who draw this kind of picture and have this psychological perspective have a better survival rate than people who draw negative-looking pictures.

FIGURE 50

This woman wrote "Help" on her belly after taking my advice to patients who are going into the hospital. I always tell them to bring a Siegel Kit. It has a felt-tip marker, a noisemaker, and a water gun. The felt-tip marker is for writing "Cut here" and "Not this one, stupid." One woman wrote just above her pubic hair: "Don't mow the lawn." With patient humor like this, everybody in the operating room laughs and becomes family. The noisemaker can save lives. One woman was choking on her food in the hospital, and when she pushed the call button, no one responded. She told me later: "If I hadn't had a roommate, I'd be dead." The water gun is to drench those who disturb your privacy for no good reason.

FIGURE 51

Purple is a spiritual color, and although the use of purple can suggest a person is dying, I don't think the color of this patient's chemotherapy indicates that she believes it's going to kill her. I think she sees that it can heal her. The red spots on her body — an emotional color

— signify the cancer. The fewer white spots among them, which are practically invisible, are her white cells. This patient's perception of herself as a stick figure is not very empowering. She has drawn herself in black and is honest enough to show that she is unhappy. But because nobody is shown administering the chemotherapy, and because she has colored it purple, she appears to feel the treatment is more of a gift from God. Her feet are turned toward it, showing that her intuition believes it will be helpful to her.

As far as treatment is concerned, I would say to her, "Yes, go ahead and give it a try because of the way you look in this drawing, the color of the treatment, and the direction of your feet." I would also point out to her that the cancer appears at multiple sites and is red, showing that it is creating an emotional issue in her life. How people visualize themselves matters: if they show a thousand cancer cells and few white cells, then what's going on in their bodies will match this. I would recommend to this patient that she change her image of, and belief about, herself.

FIGURE 52

This woman's chemotherapy is delivered with a black syringe, and she's not allowing it into her body. Her eyes and mouth are black, and the cancer spots look purple, and in this case the purple appears to represent death. Her message seems to be: "This is going to kill me. My disease is going to turn me into a spirit." She doesn't have a nose for inspiration, so she cannot breathe life in, which suggests she feels her treatment is not life enhancing. One foot is turned to her right, the west, the place of darkness, and her shoes are black.

She also looks as if she's fading away: her upper body is light pink (suggesting covered-up emotion and pain), and she's showing her mastectomy scars. Susan Bach notes that sick children may initially draw outdoor scenes in healthy, vivid colors like green, and then, over time, the color in their next drawings may become lighter and lighter, sometimes because the artists apply less pressure to the page; sometimes because they choose paler shades. When this happens, says Bach, it indicates that the light of life is fading, is leaving them. Similarly, the picture this woman has drawn does not bode well for her future.

FIGURE 53

This dramatic drawing has a lot of color. Since the patient has left her feet out of the picture, I'd say she was feeling stuck at the time she drew it. And she *was* stuck, because she was about sixteen years old and her parents had taken her power away. They had made her get chemotherapy against her will, until finally she refused to continue. When they brought her to my office, they wanted me to convince their daughter to take further treatment. I asked her to draw me a picture. When I saw the words *I hate you*, I asked whether that meant she hated cancer. She said, "No, I don't hate the cancer; the cancer is going through the same hell I'm going through. It's crying and saying, 'Help me.'"

What a statement; she was feeling sorry for the cancer! Who did she want to stick the spear into, then? "I want to stick it into my doctor," she told me. "He made my bald, ugly head and my horrible knee." So her anger was focused on the doctors. I don't know how her case concluded, but at least the parents gained a better understanding of where she was coming from. I suggested they give their daughter back her power and let her decide what to do.

The word *patient* is derived from a word meaning "submissive sufferer." This implies that if you're a "good" patient, you'll endure suffering, surgery, and deformation of the body, plus any complications that happen, all without expressing anger. And perhaps you'll die on a schedule that pleases everyone, or die from medical decisions made by professionals who do not know you as a person and give you the wrong treatment.

I tell people not to be good patients, but to be respants instead. What is a respant? It means you are a "responsible participant." You take responsibility for your treatment. The doctor may prescribe something, but *you* are the one who decides whether to do it. And when you make decisions, you don't judge yourself as a failure if the result is not the one you were hoping for. The way I put it is: Are you trying not to die, or to do what is right for *you?*

Most people go through difficult procedures in the hope they will not die, or will live longer, but some are more concerned about the quality of life and will choose a treatment that they can live with, even if it means they may not live as long. A respant decides what is right for him; and if it doesn't work, he doesn't get mad at himself, thinking he's a failure. When people say, "I don't want to die," I tell them "then do everything your doctor recommends; if it doesn't work, at least you won't feel guilty for not trying."

FIGURE 54

The teenage boy in this picture is lying on his hospital bed getting chemotherapy. I think he probably feels it is good for him, because he has colored it orange, the color that signifies change. But he's not letting it flow into his body; it stops at his wrist. Under the bed is a vomit basin for the side effects he anticipates. The IV pole is black, and he's outlined himself in black, so he's feeling a lot of grief about the cancer. The window is black too, but there are blue clouds (life energy) in the window, and the blue clouds are a good sign. His clothing is blue, as well, although that may simply be the color of the hospital gown, in which case it has no significance. The yellow of the mattress he's lying on is a positive color if it relates to his treatment.

The thing that troubles me is the doorway on the right: what the boy needs is company. The family decided he should have chemotherapy, and he went to the hospital to get it. But where's the family? They're not there to support him. He's lying there all by himself, suffering the consequences of their decision without their presence and love.

Try this experiment: Put your hand in a bucket of ice while sitting alone in the bathroom. Keep track of the elapsing time. Write down how long it takes before it becomes too painful and you have to pull your hand out of the ice. Then take the bucket of ice into the living room and get your whole family and all your pets to sit around you. Put your hand back in the bucket of ice, and watch how much longer you can tolerate it when surrounded by the people who love you. This neatly illustrates how important love and company are to people who are struggling to become well.

FIGURES 55 AND 56

This woman drew herself in a box that has a strap to hold her head still while the radiation is directed to her tumor (fig. 55). The line forming one side of the bed goes over her foot, so she can't get out. Symbolically she's boxed in, and the fact that she has no fingers in the drawing suggests she's not getting a grip on things. She doesn't have a nose, implying her lack of inspiration about the treatment. A similar lack of emotional support and nourishment is suggested by her technicians, who also lack noses and are standing on the other side of the window, completely separated from her.

In figure 56, the radiation rays are red and black, two strong emotional colors, so she is going to have a lot of reaction to the treatment. Notice that she has aimed the treatment not only at the tumor, which is depicted as a large black spot on her jaw, but also at her shoulder, neck, and face. One nice thing is that the black tumor cells are surrounded by her immune system, which is a nurturing earth color. This brown area looks almost as if it's made up of bricks or marbles that are blocking the tumor off and confining it to that area. This is a helpful approach, but nevertheless I think she's going to have innumerable side effects where the arrows are pointing because of her attitude toward it.

FIGURE 57

Here the patient is lying on the operating table; his cardiogram is on the wall, and he has two intravenous lines attached to him. The green sheet draping over him is a healthy color, but no one is there to take care of the guy. It looks as if he died and somebody covered his dead body. Most likely this patient is fearful about going into the operating room, because he's displaying his cardiogram and it's black. The cardiogram may suggest that he feels nobody is watching over him, and that his heart may stop as a result, and so he's scared to death.

FIGURE 58

In this drawing, you see the opposite of fear. What a difference. Because she feels that love and God are in the operating room, this woman is not going to have any trouble. The table is sunshine yellow, and rays of life-giving energy surround her. The surgeon is not wearing a mask and gown or gloves — he's there for her as a person, touching her, relating to her as a human being. The surgeon has a rainbow over his head and the patient is imagining a flower; each of these is connected to the person by four bubbles. Four is the number for completeness or wholeness; it may also mean something personal to the artist. Three hearts and three purple musical notes dance in the air. Three could refer to the Trinity. There are twelve flowers, which may signify a period of time, people, or some other personal meaning. It's just beautiful. This is all peaceful, healing imagery. I would not worry about this patient at all.

FIGURE 59

This man is hiding his hands and has no feet; he's cut off. How can he help himself — how can he reach out to do what he needs to do? It's nice that his shoulders are rounded, because problems will slide off. The man shows two big scars on his chest and yet thinks of the disease as being outside his body, as if he can't do anything about it. He has eyes, nose, ear, and a mouth, but if you have drawn your disease outside your body, it says you haven't accepted the reality of it, or the responsibility for dealing with it, so how can you have an effect on it?

His intuitive wisdom is telling us what is going on in his body. Here the black cells are cancer cells, the treatment is red, and his white cells are like yellow Pac-Men. One cancer cell at the bottom is not affected by the treatment, so I'd say that 80 percent of the cancer is being addressed by the treatment and by his immune system.

Using the same metaphors he chose for his drawing, I would say to him, "Get your hands out, get your feet going, and accept the disease as being in your body." Acceptance doesn't mean he's facing a bad outcome; it's about realizing: "Okay, this has happened, and I need to participate in what's going on, not just stand there." We've got to get him to improve the imagery in his visualization sessions and to see 100 percent of his cancer being affected.

FIGURE 60

This man has used horses to represent his white cells. I'd say to him, "Don't limit yourself to seven horses; use a hundred or more." (One woman used popcorn — that's a good image. The kernels have high energy and seemingly endless numbers, and as they pop open they can smother the cancer cells.) In this drawing the chemotherapy drug is not affecting all of the man's cancer cells. I'd ask him to visualize it so that *all* the cancer cells are under attack, and I'd suggest that he visualize this happening *inside* the body.

FAMILY: THE FIRST SUPPORT SYSTEM

FIGURE 61

A tree is symbolic of the family or of a person. The trunk represents the body; the upper part of a tree signifies consciousness, and the roots are what's beneath the surface — the past and the unconscious. Here, all you see is the body portion of the tree, and there's a hole in the heart of it. The picture was drawn in pencil, with no color, leaving out emotions and life. When the members of a family aren't communicating, all the life goes out of the family. The father has his hands in his pockets. The daughter is reaching out to the mother, but the mother is not reciprocating, and no one is touching the boy. They need to communicate, support each other, and talk about their feelings.

Figure 62

Look at the sofa. Even though there's an empty seat there, this child is sitting by herself. She drew herself in purple, so I knew she was telling me: "I am going to die of my disease. I'm going to become a spirit." I showed this picture to the parents, and it had a profound impact on the whole family. A year or so after she died, they called me and said, "Thank you for your help with that drawing, because we devoted a lot more time to her. We had a wonderful relationship with her and healed all our lives before she died." So the process of her dying was not just about losing or failing but instead brought them a sense of fulfillment, and it meant a great deal to them that their daughter could die feeling so loved.

Figure 63

The black roof on this house could be the actual color, or it could signify the artist's emotional issues. Before you interpret a drawing like this one, it's important to ask, "What color is the roof of the house you live in?" I once had a patient draw a red house and black car. As it turned out, these two emotional colors signaled that her husband was an alcoholic who smoked in the house and drove while intoxicated, making it dangerous for her to be in the house or car with him. Here, two individuals are sitting together in front of the house, and it's obvious that there's room for both of them in it. There's also a dog and flowers, and the entire page is filled in. When people fill in their pictures, it says that their lives are full. The chimneys give the hot air an easy escape from this house. When these two people have a problem, they're going to resolve it. It's not going to build up pressure and destroy their home life.

Figure 64

The butterfly is a symbol of transformation, so change is going on in the lives of the people in this drawing. This butterfly is purple, but it's not flying in the upper left corner, where the death concept is represented.

And the drawing is not a tragic picture, so I don't see it as predictive of death. Since the butterfly occupies the middle right (the present), I see it as a symbol of spiritual transformation and change — it relates to what is happening in the family now. Above them is a rainbow with the colors in proper order, so it expresses the idea of order in this family's life and a sense of wholeness. They are touching each other, and there's color everywhere; the picture is full of life. The four flowers could represent the people. Three flowers are closer together and one stands a little farther away, like the little boy, but you get the feeling of energy, growth, and healthy relationships, and so it feels good to look at the picture.

FIGURE 65

The number seven appears in the center of this picture, so it could be the age of the person who drew it. There are many rays of sunshine in the upper right quadrant, representing the present, the here and now, which could relate to the artist's life in general, people in her life, and so forth. She has included four clouds, but they're blue — a positive, healthy color — not black. There are also three waves. It would be useful to talk with her about all those numbers. What's particularly interesting is that the four clouds and three waves add up to seven, so I'd ask her about this as well. The number seven, which is also the number of days in a week, could be about the artist's life situation and what the change is creating. This picture was drawn by an adopted child, and I would point out to the family: "She shows that you're in the same boat, but you are at opposite ends of the boat. The arms of each person are reaching out, but they're not touching the other person, and she needs you to be closer to her."

FIGURES 66 AND 67

These were drawn by a doctor friend after an auto accident that she was lucky to survive. Her car had gone off the road, and fortunately somebody noticed it, found her, and rescued her. But she became paraplegic as a result of the accident. In figure 66, where she's alone, you see her on a path curving downhill. There's still some sunshine in her life, but there are also clouds with some emotion in them — she's added a little red to them. They are not black clouds, however, and she wears a smile, an honest one. But she has a big black hole in her heart — that's her wound: her paralysis. Imagine — she was going to be a doctor, and look what happened to her while she was in medical school. She found it hard to get the school to accept her back, because of her paraplegia.

In the picture she drew of herself with her boyfriend (fig. 67), she's whole. As I mentioned before, when loved ones are around, pain and problems of all kinds diminish. Her path is not going downhill anymore and now it's green. When somebody loves you, your path in life becomes a healing one; it becomes a different story when you're together. She feels complete again; she's standing. They're looking at each other and holding hands. The four flowers could be other people, or they might represent time, possibly the number of years before she completes her medical training.

Figure 68

This was drawn by a nun. She's the person on the far left, the one with the cancer. She said, "I need more help from my family," and then she handed this picture to me. I pointed out that her family has a genetic defect: their arms and hands are fixed to their bodies. The blue dress of the woman in the middle has lines crossing her hands, so they're tied down and she can't use them. The hands of the others are tucked in pockets or stuck to their sides. Nobody's really touching, although the brothers are brushing against each other. The third brother from the right is stepping on another brother's toes. Things like that sneak into the drawings, and they are not accidental. There is something going on between those two guys — given the symbolism of one stepping on the other's toes and the way their bodies are situated. The two are signaling that they are just not open to each other.

At the bottom, "My family" is written in a reddish color, though faint, showing that passion and affection just aren't there. I told my patient she would have to reach out and ask for help. That's survival behavior. If this patient is being too nice to ask her family for help, she's hurting herself. She must get help from them or turn to another resource.

FIGURE 69

I'm sure this was drawn by one of our kids. When he drew me, one of my arms was longer than the other from carrying my briefcase; I was always off to the hospital doing something, and he is expressing emotion about that. Bobbie has a black outfit but it doesn't represent illness; it's what she was wearing when she posed for this picture. Stephen went to law school eventually, but first he went to automotive and diesel school and was always rebuilding cars, so that's a mechanic's tool in his hands. Family members are all touching each other. Keith (on the right) has really long arms, so it could be that he's needier or is reaching out for things. But here, too, look at the broad shoulders on him, which signal that a person is taking on too much. Carolyn (in a blue sweater) and Keith are twins; in the back are John (with glasses) and Jeffrey. The trees in the background look healthy.

Encouraging your kids to make drawings is a great way to open discussion about things they feel uncomfortable talking about. When these things show up in the pictures, the kids can discuss them. When I'd visit the school on parent days, my kids' teachers were often amazed that I could look at the other students' drawings and tell them about the children's families. I might see that the family was undergoing divorce, illness, or one of many other different things, and the teachers would ask, "How do you know that?" I'd say, "It's in the picture."

Our kids learned to use drawings as life tools. They were aware that I knew a lot about drawings, so if they were trying to make a decision about something and drew a picture about it, and I walked into the room, they had no problem asking for my help. But if they were working on a drawing about something personal and I walked in, they'd cover it with an object or slump over to hide it. They didn't want me interpreting those drawings and worrying about them or prying into their private lives.

FIGURE 70

Wanting to make a decision about whether to remain where she was living or to move closer to her family prompted this drawing. What do you think she decided?

DOCTOR'S R_x
FOR PARENTS AND OTHER FAMILY MEMBERS

Put out some white paper and a box of crayons, and then ask your kids to draw a self-portrait, followed by a family picture, for you to display on the refrigerator. Don't tell them these are for you to analyze. You will be amazed to see how your kids talk to you through their drawings. Use the drawings as another way of getting closer to a family member and helping to heal family wounds through your new insights. When family members have a decision to make, you can then tell them to draw their various choices to help give them insights into which choice is best for them — whether the decision is about which treatment is best, where to go to college, who to marry, where to live, or something else.

Chapter 7

ANIMALS, PSYCHICS, AND INTUITIVES

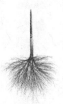

There is no conclusion in infinity. There is only inclusion....
We arrive at the same non-arrivable place that We never left.

— GLORIA WENDROFF

I believe we are here to contribute love to the planet, each of us in our own way. And while our human contribution to love is essential, humans are not the planet's only source of love. When someone who lives alone tells me he is suffering because of an illness, grief, or depression, I advise him to develop a relationship. When you give meaning to your life in this way, it changes your life and how you and your body feel. My prescription for those who are ailing is to bring other living things into their lives, other beings who depend on them and that they feel connected to, such as a dog or cat. When people do this, they feel as if they must not die and break the animal's heart. By opening your heart to an animal's love, you give your body a reason to live.

Studies have revealed the survival benefits of having a dog, cat, or fish in your home or in nursing homes — and even of having plants, when the nursing home residents are given responsibility for care of the plants. Other studies found that, twelve months after suffering a heart attack, patients who came from homes with a dog had a significantly lower mortality rate than patients whose homes had no dog. In another study, stockbrokers with hypertension received treatment, but half of them also received a dog to take home and to work. Those with the dog maintained lower blood pressure.

One of my patients with cancer had twelve cats, and her family was concerned that her home wasn't clean. They had even stopped visiting her there, because of the odor. They also worried that caring for the animals would be too much for her during the weeks of treatment, and they told me they had convinced my patient to let them give her cats away. I said to the family, "If you take the cats away from her, she's dead. Tell her you can't find a home for them; then go in and clean up the place." They left the cats with her; the cats became her therapy, and she went on to have a successful recovery.

Our internal environment changes when emotions spark a series of electrical and chemical reactions. When a person strokes an animal, the hormone oxytocin is released into the blood of each. This is the same hormone that flows through a mother's body after childbirth and causes her to bond with the baby. When the father and other family members hold the infant, they receive a similar burst of the bonding chemical. Hormones and neurotransmitters that help us relate to people and other living beings send live messages throughout our bodies. A simpler way of saying it is: bonding and caring is good for your health.

Not only do you have receptors in your brain, but you also have them in your stomach, fingertips, and many other places throughout the body. Why do people say they "feel good all over," or that they have a "gut feeling" or a "broken heart?" When internal chemicals bond with receptors, your whole body becomes the beneficiary or suffers the consequences, depending on which hormones have been released. I'm talking about your bone marrow, the lining of your blood vessels, every organ, and every cell inside you.

The adage about animals stealing center stage is based on the fact that they have a wonderful way of making us laugh. Who can be miserable when her dog chases its tail, or her kitten jumps in fright as it walks by a mirror and sees its reflection? Science has proven that the composition of hormones and neuropeptides circulating in the blood of the individual who laughs several times a day differs from that of the person who is depressed, angry, or fearful; the person who laughs also has better survival statistics.

I cannot count the number of times I have seen the beneficial effect of an animal's love on a patient's will to live and that person's resultant recovery. The message we need to learn from animals is this: use animals as your role models. Go outside and exercise. Play as often as you can. Make close bonds and friendships while practicing nonjudgmental listening, and show an empathic heart. Care for yourself as well as you care for your pets. Please don't do what one cat lover did. She and her husband stopped smoking in the house and moved their unhealthy habit to the backyard in order not to kill their cats with secondhand smoke. If you want to live and be there for your pets, love yourself as much as you love them, and quit the unhealthy addictions.

DOCTOR'S R_x

Take a dog for a walk. Notice how you feel while walking with your canine companion as opposed to walking unaccompanied. Do people around you behave differently? For example, do they stop and talk with you? (A large percentage of the women interviewed in one city said they met the man they married while walking their dogs.) After the walk, pay attention to your mood. How does it compare to the way you felt before you walked the dog? If you are not ambulatory, have someone take you to an animal sanctuary. Hold a cat, small dog, or rabbit in your lap and spend time stroking it. Notice how you feel before, during, and after. Volunteer to go again.

IT ALL COMES AROUND

Animals can act as catalysts, providing beneficial effects in our lives when we're mired in challenging circumstances. In *A Book of Miracles*, Mary Rose Anderson tells of rescuing a stray cat that saved her daughter. Frances had been diagnosed with oppositional defiant disorder and Tourette's syndrome, and she had major learning disabilities. Mary Rose compared her daughter's daily tantrums and defiant behavior to that of the young Helen Keller before Annie Sullivan entered her life. It seemed to Mary Rose as though no one would ever be able to reach her daughter, regardless of the dedicated people trying to help her.

"When Harry the Child Whisperer entered our home," says Mary Rose, "I watched in amazement as my daughter began to change."[1] Harry assigned himself the role of constant companion to Frances, and he purred with nonjudgmental love as he watched every move she made. Prior to Harry's adoption, Frances had frequent loud eruptions of emotion and refused to focus during tutoring sessions or fell into silent defiance. But with the tail-swishing cat sitting on the chair beside her, Frances became more focused on the task at hand. She discussed whatever she was doing with Harry, engaging him in her lessons. Every night, no matter what had happened during the day, Harry climbed into bed with Frances and loved her to sleep. Under the calming influence of the rescued cat, Frances grew from a child with little hope of ever progressing, into a happy, productive young woman who loves to write poetry. This is an excerpt from one of her poems:

> What if I were my cat?
> I wonder what it would be like to always wake me up at seven
> chewing on my toes. Do my toes taste good?
> I wonder what it would be like to put my feline face

one inch from my PATIENT, LOVING owner...

and meow.

Would I like hearing the sound of my own voice?[2]

Horses too play a significant therapeutic role for people with physical, mental, developmental, and emotional challenges. Individuals who undergo hippotherapy (horse therapy) look forward all week to that day, no matter if they have suffered a stroke, have undergone amputation, or have autism, Down syndrome, cerebral palsy, post–traumatic stress disorder, or any other condition that makes life uniquely challenging.

Gail Corell, president and volunteer coordinator for the Equestrian Crossings therapeutic riding program, believes that the physical and psychological improvements she has seen in their riders borders on the miraculous. "A horse reaches out to the heart of somebody in a way that no therapy ball could," says Gail. She told me a story about Kirbey, their Percheron therapy horse that was originally rescued from a circus and then, later, rescued by the program's instructor from a neglectful owner. "Last week, we took Kirbey to the South Whidbey Island Children's Festival," said Gail. "While standing in our section of the fairground, Kirbey directed his attention to something at the far end of the field. His behavior and body language signaled to our licensed vaulting coach and riding instructor, Miriam Burk, that he was keen to go over there. Wondering what had caught his interest with such intensity, she mounted the horse and let him take the lead. Kirbey strode out purposefully through that throng of people, passing hundreds of children and parents. He adores children," explained Gail, "and passing by their outstretched hands was not something he usually wants to do. At the opposite end of the field, a girl was seated in a wheelchair, and she was all by herself. Kirbey walked directly up to her, stopped, and then lowered his head, letting her stroke him while their eyes [engaged in] a long, soulful conversation. From the moment that horse set eyes on the girl, Kirbey knew exactly what she needed and he brought it to her."[3]

Emily Brink, a physical therapist and therapeutic riding instructor at Equestrian Crossings, has seen wheelchair-bound students who had been unable to hold themselves upright without assistance improve to such a degree that, in only eight months, they could sit upright and control their head movements. "In the hospital outpatient clinic," says Emily, "I'm lucky to get a patient to move their pelvis between thirty and sixty repetitions per session. But when someone is sitting on a horse's back, the horse's movement forces the rider's body to make movements that mimic walking, and the rider's pelvis will be making repetitions well up into the thousands. This stimulates their brain and sends wonderful input to the core muscles; it improves posture and balance, develops coordination, and increases head and neck control. The rider's self-confidence and overall mood get a tremendous boost. This sparks growth and development on multiple levels, making an incredible, positive change in their lives."[4]

Animals communicate through consciousness rather than words, and they have much to teach us about being complete. In *No Buddy Left Behind: Bringing U.S. Troops' Dogs and Cats Safely Home from the Combat Zone*, Terri Crisp tells her story of the first eight months of Operation Baghdad Pups. Stray animals who had adopted American soldiers in the war zone had become family to the troops, and when their soldier buddies were redeployed, the animals needed a miracle to get out of Iraq. One Special Forces soldier returned home after several years of deployments, unable to speak to anyone and suffering severe symptoms of post–traumatic stress disorder. His mother feared she had lost her son. When she learned about the dog he'd left behind, she contacted the organization and begged for help. With their intervention, her son's war buddy was eventually rescued and brought home to him in the States. When this mother looked out the window and saw her son talking to the dog, with his arm around the animal's shoulders, and the dog listening to his every word, she cried tears of relief. The soldier's mother said, "The war took my son away, but that dog saved his life and brought my son back again."[5]

Crisp also tells the story of an officer in the U.S. Air Force who worked on a mental health team in Baghdad, and who rescued a puppy from the streets. Soldiers had been reluctant to come to the center for much-needed counseling, but when the puppy joined the counselors, soldiers came to the station and asked to see him. "While holding the dog, they would suddenly open up, and we could establish a therapeutic relationship," the officer explains. "He was the best health technician on the team!" After being saved by Operation Baghdad Pups, the puppy, named Patton, was brought to the States, where he lived with the retiring officer. Months after the officer's return, she discovered she had breast cancer. "Patton became my therapy and my coach. I don't know what I would have done without him. He made me laugh and gave me hope. Now I'm well again and training to run a marathon."[6]

Service animals have played an invaluable role in helping people to adapt and achieve things that most of us take for granted. When Jacquei shared her story with me, I was fascinated to learn that she was one of the first female mechanics to work on fighter jets for the U.S. Navy. She specialized in ejector seats, oxygen systems, fire extinguishers, and other lifesaving systems, and during her five years with the Blue Angels she went on tour across the United States and Canada. Jacquei's favorite days were Fridays, when the Blue Angels put on shows for kids associated with the Make-A-Wish Foundation or they visited schools. "I loved it because the kids are curious and genuinely interested," she said. "They asked good questions too, like why pilots don't fall out of the jet when they fly upside down." Jacquei had firsthand experience that helped her to answer that question. Her reenlistment was officiated by a naval officer as she rode in the back of an F/A-18 Hornet — inverted — only two hundred feet off the water.

Jacquei was forced to retire from the U.S. Navy for medical reasons. Her most debilitating injury was not the physical injuries incurred on duty but the severe post–traumatic stress disorder that haunted her daily life. "It's like a light switch that suddenly turns on, and you can't turn it off," Jacquei explained. "An unexpected noise or movement puts me into a hyperalert state, and then a hairpin trigger shoots me into panic, fear, anger, or rage." Jacquei suffers typical symptoms: sleep disturbances such as nightmares and sleepwalking, memory loss, startle response, and giant mood swings. Medication has not been successful in controlling all her symptoms.

"That's where Sampson comes in," she said as she stroked her four-pound Chihuahua service dog. "He knows before I do that something in my body is going wrong. He'll climb into my lap, put his paws on my shoulders, and lick my face until I pay attention to him, drawing my focus away from the source of my agitation. Just looking at him and feeling him touch me calms the panic before it takes over. Some people scoff when I say this mini Chihuahua is a service dog, but Sampson has a Rottweiler spirit and protects me no matter where I go. His strong sense of duty to me makes it possible for me to go out in the world and live a relatively normal life. I tell the doubters that Sampson may be small, but every day he proves that size doesn't matter."

Animals are God's complete creations, while humans are not complete. If you are suffering, bring an animal into your life. Love the animal and care for it. You will find that love given becomes love received, and that the reward of giving love is well-being.

PSYCHIC COMMUNICATION

I believe that creation comes from loving, conscious, intelligent energy, and when we leave our bodies in a near-death experience, we become un-alive again and reenter that state of perfection from which we came. I believe the intelligence that remains when we have a near-death experience, or when we find ourselves hovering above our bodies, is the same force that communicates via our dreams, speaks through symbols to our intuition, and guides our inner knowing. This, the universal collective consciousness, is the source of all creation, and it communicates with our consciousness.

Consciousness is nonlocal, which means it is not dependent on physical bodies, and it travels vast distances in an instant while crossing boundaries of language, species, space, and time. Amelia Kinkade, author, psychic, and animal communicator, told me while she was sitting in Los Angeles where to find our cat, Boo Boo, who had disappeared from our son's home in Connecticut. While "seeing" through the cat's eyes, she described the house and yard in incredible detail, and she identified where the cat was hiding. I went out and rescued Boo Boo from the exact place Amelia had seen from almost three thousand miles away.

Amelia also taught me that I had to quiet my mind in order to be able to communicate with my animals. One of my biggest problems is my tendency to mentally go to a place of fear when one of our pets is missing or acting strangely. I try to force them to do my will, and I bellow in fear or anger as I call their names while searching for them, or I go into my head and decide what the animal is thinking, neither of which ever works.

When Amelia referred to animal communication, she was talking not about verbal sounds or physical touch but about connecting my consciousness with the frequency of consciousness that the animals' intelligence tunes into and understands. We are all capable of making this connection, but before nonlocal intelligence can communicate with us, we have to enter a state of mental stillness. It cannot get through when we are in turmoil, because turbulent minds cannot achieve the quiet state that reflects mirror images.

I have had many experiences when a voice has spoken to me, and it has usually happened while I was taking a walk or otherwise exercising and my mind was quiet. One such event happened just after I published a book called *Buddy's Candle*. It is a story about a little boy's love for his dog, Buddy, and how the dog taught him to appreciate life and handle death.[7] I had written the story to help people of all ages deal with the loss of a loved one of any species.

On a Saturday morning, after the first printed copies of *Buddy's Candle* arrived on my doorstep, I took our dog, Furphy, out for a walk. In the quietness, I heard a voice say to me, "Go to the animal shelter." I have learned from experience to always listen to this voice, and I feel it is coming from God or, as my wife Bobbie says, from God-knows-where.

I decided to bring some copies of the book to the shelter, and when I arrived with Furphy I found a volunteer sitting next to the door holding a dog. The voice almost seemed as if it spoke through me as I said, "What's his name?"

"His name is Buddy," she replied. "A woman brought him in less than fifteen minutes ago because she doesn't like how he behaves."

The coincidence of his name struck me, and her comment about his owner reminded me of the only dog I had in my childhood. My mother, who did not want an animal in the house, would lower him by his harness out the window until he peed, then haul him back in again. After only a week, when I came home from school she told me that my dog was sick and that they had returned him.

How could I not adopt this animal? I knew that the collective consciousness had made the decision for me. His color matched Furphy's coat, and he had no tail. Furphy's had been amputated, so they matched. It was obvious we were family. At least in this case I got to choose my relatives. I gave everyone at the shelter a copy of *Buddy's Candle* and took Buddy home with me.

Synchronous events, circumstances, names, numbers, and so on are signposts that a greater intelligence is playing a guiding role in the way those events happen. Remember, there are no coincidences, and our unconscious is always creating our future.

Months later I was at the shelter again, and they told me a dog named Simon, my dad's name, was there and that he needed surgery to remove a large tumor. My background as an oncology surgeon made me aware of the urgency of his situation, so I helped pay his medical bills and took him home too. After he was fully recovered, we found a family who would give him lots of love and would keep sharing his story with us. We now have a cat named Simon, and I no longer reveal our family names to the people at the shelter.

Communicating with animals is inherent in all of us, Amelia

explains in her book *The Language of Miracles*.[8] Thought and emotion are electromagnetic waves that travel in specific frequencies, just like radio waves. If you are completely still when an animal sends out a thought or feeling, you can learn to match the frequency of your thought and emotion to the animal's and vibrate on his wave. Animals think in pictures; they experience a broad scope of emotions and possess a huge capacity to love, give, and have meaningful relationships. When they realize that we have heard and understood their feelings and thoughts, they are grateful and reward us with their own better health and their devotion to us.

My animals also know what day I plan to groom them and make it hard for me to find them. Two outdoor cats didn't show up for a week after I made their vet appointment, which I'd scheduled for the early morning with the idea that I could catch them and take them to the vet when they showed up for breakfast. The morning after I cancelled their appointment, they showed up bright and early for breakfast.

Now that I'm a believer, when I am presented with an animal problem I ask myself the WWAD question: What would Amelia do? Our beloved house rabbit, Smudge Eliza-Bunny, always began her day by running out the pet door in the morning, and she'd stay in our fenced-in front yard all day with our other creatures. I always wanted to know why she would allow my wife to pick her up and bring her into the house in the evening without any problem, but would run around for ten or fifteen minutes before letting me catch her when I attempted to do it. Most evenings, I was the one to bring her in, so it bothered me that Smudge made my gatekeeping job so difficult.

So after learning about animal communication from Amelia, my first WWAD was to go into our front yard the next evening and, in my head, ask our rabbit, "Smudge, why don't you let me pick you up and bring you inside the way you let Bobbie do it?"

When I get an unexpected answer in my mind, it verifies for me that it is coming from the animal and not my imagination. In this case the answer was: *You don't treat the cats that way.* When I went on to ask what she meant by that, Smudge communicated that I didn't make the cats come in at a specific time. Instead I gave them the freedom to go in and out until my bedtime. I explained to Smudge that cats could defend themselves should a predator get into the yard, but I was worried about her being out late when it grew dark.

After our communication, Smudge hopped over and let me pick her up, and she continued to do so every day afterward. I will admit, some days she would smile at me and remind me of the old days for a minute or two, but I could tell it was just her sense of humor. And when I had appointments, I would go out into the yard, tell her I needed to leave the house and that I would feel better if she would come in. She always hopped right over to me when she knew I had a schedule to keep.

When Smudge died, Amelia said, "She will be with Rose, who loves her." Amelia didn't know that my mom's name was Rose, or that Mom would die shortly after Smudge's death. Now I know they are together again, sharing stories about me.

Last year I went shopping with our two dogs, Furphy and Buddy. The car we got into was a new minivan with remote control door mechanisms on the key. After shopping, I returned to the car and was horrified to see the side door was wide open, owing to my accidentally hitting the control. Buddy, the one I worried about most because he used to be terrified of going in the car, was sitting in the car peacefully, while Furphy was nowhere to be seen. My first reaction was panic, and I began to run around calling out his name and searching the areas around the parking lot. Then I remembered, "You are not doing what Amelia taught you," and so I asked myself, WWAD?

I quieted down and went into Furphy's head to find out what he was thinking. Immediately I realized he was searching for me, and he was probably at the front desk of the market, with someone asking over the loud speaker: "Whose dog is this?" I say that because, when I attended Amelia's workshop at the Omega Institute, Furphy was not let into the dining hall. So during the lunch break, I left him at the back door and told him to wait for me to come out, which he usually does.

But that time he didn't. Before long, a man came through the hall with Furphy in his arms, asking whose dog it was, and we were reunited. Apparently Furphy had run around to the front door and into the foyer, searching for me. He won over everyone's heart, and they let him stay.

This time, as I approached the front entrance of the supermarket, I saw a security guard sitting in his car. He lowered the driver's window and asked, "Are you looking for a dog?" I answered yes, and he said, "Here he is, on the front seat with air conditioning, water, and treats." The guard went on to tell me that he had seen Furphy walking toward the front of the market and didn't want him to be hit by a car, so he had picked him up and kept him safe. After I thanked the man, Furphy followed me back to the car, and we have never had that problem again.

Now to explain about Buddy and why I was surprised at who stayed in the car and who left: After adopting Buddy from the animal shelter, I could never get him to go into a car without difficulty. He even jumped out of the car once when I stopped for gas. At home, if I didn't have him on a leash, getting him into the car was a frustrating, time-consuming experience. Finally one day I thought, WWAD?

I then calmed myself and asked Buddy why he wouldn't get in the car. I was amazed at his answer. He said the woman who previously owned him was very nice, but when her husband came home from work she would ask him to take the dog for a walk. Buddy told me, *He would put me in the car and then drive to a bar and leave me in the car. When he came out he would be abusive because of his drinking and just take me home, never having let me out for a walk. So getting into a car reminds me of all the abuse I received, and it scares me.*

On that day, Buddy's disobedience ended. We now understood each other. Buddy can enjoy the car because he knows we are always going out to share the day. He loves to chase moving things in the woods near our home, and yet I never have to worry about his not coming home. Whenever I open the side door of the car, before I can say, "Jumpee upee!" he is in the front seat raring to go.

Furphy and Buddy are my cotherapists in support groups and

anywhere they are allowed entry. The only problem is, now that they know we can communicate, Furphy never stops telling me what to do and interrupts therapy groups unless he gets a treat, which is my sign to him that we are starting the therapy session.

The other day I drove off, thinking they were both in the car, but after a half mile I realized no one was telling me where to go or what to do. I turned to look in the back of the car and saw only Buddy. I immediately connected with Furphy and told him I was sorry and was coming home. I turned around and drove, knowing Furphy would be sitting in the driveway giving me that *Boy, are you a dumbbell* look that God's complete creations give to us incomplete human beings. It's a look I also used to get from the cats when I accidentally locked them out overnight. Now, every evening before I get into bed, I take attendance, intuitively and physically, to be sure all our kids are in the house and no one is locked out. I let them know I want them in for their protection and not just because I desire their company, and that's when they show up at the door.

My friend experienced an intuitive connection with her dog while she was attending an animal healing workshop and her dog had been left at home. Cindy wrote,

During our meditation session it blew my mind when unexpectedly I found myself looking up at someone who seemed as tall as a giant. I was at the level of her knees. I suddenly realized the giant was me, and I was no longer in my body! Being a short person, I had never thought of myself as tall. That's when it hit me that I was not looking through my own eyes, but seeing from my dog's perspective. I could understand Pickles's thoughts and feel his feelings. The love he had for me was so encompassing, I was almost overwhelmed. I have never experienced a depth of pure love such as that. Its existence was more than heart and a feeling; it was his soul radiating for me, and it nearly brought me to tears.

Pickles had stopped using his back leg after two consecutive knee operations. During recovery from the first surgery, he'd managed to remove the cone collar, pull out his stitches, and lick it, and the resultant infection damaged the area to the point that he had to have a second surgery. Weeks after the wound healed, he would not use that leg but let it hang limp while the others took over. On the day of the animal healing workshop, Pickles's feelings and picture thoughts made me understand that he believed he had done something bad, and that's why his leg had been hurt. He felt really, really sorry and was trying his best to be good, so he stopped using the leg.

I felt awful when I realized how Pickles had interpreted his pain from the second operation as punishment. I assured him with my mind that he had done *nothing* wrong, that he was always a good boy and we loved him dearly. When I got home after the three-day workshop, the first thing I did was spend time with him doing energy work on his leg and body, and let him know how loved he was. I continued the routine of healing and loving sessions every day.

Immediately Pickles began to use the leg. Within two weeks, he even began to run on it, and after four weeks, when I tested his leg's resistance at extension, it had increased from about 20 percent of normal resistance to around 80 percent. What amazed me was that, not only did he lose his fear of using the leg, but he was healed in another way too. Pickles had suffered from epileptic seizures for as long as we'd had him, and the vet wanted to put him on medication to reduce their frequency. The medicine made him feel sleepy all the time. If all he wanted to do was sleep, what kind of a life was that for him? So we didn't give him the medicine. After the knee-healing sessions, Pickles never had another seizure. His epilepsy went away.

I could share many more stories about energy healing. When the vet recommended euthanizing one of our dogs because he had never seen a dog as sick as that recover, the children wouldn't let me give my consent. I saw this animal turn around completely and recover from terminal cancer with love and touch. I have experienced energy healing myself after an injury. To learn more about the topic of energy work, see *The Energy Cure*, by William Bengston, a book I have found fascinating.

CONSCIOUS HEALING ENERGY

Although I have always tried to keep an open mind, nothing in my training as a physician taught me to understand that all life-forms emit a mirror image of invisible conscious energy at the subatomic quantum level, nor that this energy can be communicated by individuals through psychic or intuitive methods. I also wasn't told that people can facilitate the spontaneous healing of physical problems in the body using conscious energy.

One day Bobbie and I were at a meeting of the American Holistic Medical Association, and the guest speaker was Olga Worrall, an author and renowned mystic who communicated with spirits and performed spiritual healings.[9] Olga said that when she worked, she tuned her personal energy field to a harmonious relationship with the universal field of energy, thus becoming a conductor between that field of energy and the patient. She explained that emanations surround every individual, and that these emanations are caused by electrical currents flowing in the physical body. She spoke of sound waves coming from the physical organs, thought waves from the mind, and vibrations from the spiritual body, or aura.

Olga's ability to channel energy had been tested by many respected scientists in dozens of controlled experiments; often the experiments took place over vast distances, so it was not about beliefs but research. I was amazed by her presentation, but because my medical training and experience did not include the possibility of what she described, I remained skeptical.

After Olga spoke, my wife said I should go up and ask her to heal my thigh injury, which had occurred while I was training to run a marathon. I told Bobbie that Olga's claims were too hard for me to believe.

So Bobbie went up and asked Olga to help me, and she came over. I sat in a chair while Olga sat in front of me and put her two hands on the injured area. Her hands felt like hot irons through my dungarees. I put my hands on my leg but didn't feel any warmth at all. Five minutes later, she was done. I stood up and walked away, totally free of any pain or problems in my leg. I have learned from events of this kind to accept what I experience as valid and not be limited by my beliefs, training, and the need to explain everything.

Olga and I became close friends after that. Years before, during a meditation, I had met my inner guide, George. I saw him as a figure with a beard, cap, and white robe. He seemed so real, but I had trouble believing that he was anything more than an element of my powerful imagination. I thought I must have pulled his character out of my subconscious.

Once, when I spoke at a funeral that Olga was attending, she came up to me and said that the whole time I was speaking to the mourners, a man was standing close beside me. She described him and his mode of dress, and it sounded exactly like the man in my meditation, the man I call George. She said he was a rabbi, which explained his clothing and cap, and she got me to understand that he was there to encourage, support, and help me to heal on this physical plane.

Another time as I was giving a lecture, I realized that the words I spoke were not mine. Someone else was deciding what was being said, and was using my voice to deliver it. A woman I had never met came up to me afterward and said, "A man was standing in front of you for the entire lecture, so I drew his picture for you." She handed me her drawing, and it was George again. That same night someone else said to me, "I have heard you speak before, but this was better than usual." Nowadays, I just leave it to George.

LIFE FOLLOWS LIFE

When the physical body dies, the individual spirit reunites with the greater consciousness but keeps its own identity. I think this also explains what we call a past-life experience, a term that describes something that happened to me. In describing it, I think of a pregnant woman carrying a child within her, one who is a different soul, but who comes from her DNA. During my past-life experience, it was as if I were being impregnated with the consciousness from another person's life, one that had been lived before mine.

I have also had many experiences in which patients who had died were still able to communicate with me or their loved ones. For example, a doctor colleague of mine, named Frank, had always been skeptical of anything that wasn't in the realm of physical science, and he didn't believe that the spirit lived on after the death of the body. A few months after Frank died, a mystic patient of mine said, "I have a message for you from someone named Frank: 'If I'd known it was this easy, I'd have bought the package a long time ago and not have resisted so much.'"

Later I called Frank's widow and gave her the message the mystic had delivered. "Oh my God, that was Frank!" she said, laughing and crying at the same time. "Whenever anyone at your group meetings brought up the topic of life after death, afterward he'd always say to me, 'I just can't buy the package.' Those were his very words."

So keep your mind open to the possibility of communication across species, time, and distance. Consider adding the work of energy practitioners to your traditional therapy or treatment. Certified practitioners of treatments such as Reiki, massage, and acupuncture often augment the healing process and affect the body in a beneficial way. Learn how to still the mental turmoil and pay attention to the voice within you. Allow the miracle of love to enter and heal your life. When we love our lives, our bodies often get the message, decide to live, and heal.

Chapter 8

LAUGH OUT LOUD

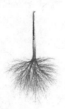

HAPPINESS

I will not give my power away
It is my happiness, mine
I create it, not you; I decide to be, not you
You can come into my happiness
But you cannot create it or destroy it
You can only enlarge it

— BERNIE SIEGEL

*L*ove and laughter are the elements we need in order to build and hold our lives together. Love makes up the bricks that we build our lives with, but what holds those bricks together? For that we need mortar, and the mortar of life is humor. I mean a childlike humor that isn't offensive and doesn't hurt anyone. The effect humor has had on my family and marriage has shown me that it's a vital force, one that enables us to create healthy relationships with other living things.

You might be asking yourself: what has laughter got to do with the art of healing? Laughter may be one of the purest of the healing arts.

What I am telling you is that laughter is one of the best therapeutic activities Mother Nature provides us with, and it doesn't cost a cent. True laughter is an outburst or expression of breath that involves the vocal cords and comes from deep in the belly. It's caused by an irresistible urge to express surprise, mirth, joy, and delight. Laughter stimulates the release of endorphins, a group of brain chemicals mentioned in an earlier chapter. These chemicals flood the body with a feel-good sensation that reaches every cell, delivering a message that says: Life is worth living, so do everything you can to survive.

Unlike the days when I was training as a physician, today we have studies documenting that cancer patients who laughed or practiced induced laughter several times a day lived longer than a control group who did not. Even so, in medical school doctors still aren't taught the value of laughter as therapy. I certainly wasn't in medical school; my patients were my teachers. They, the natives, taught me, the tourist.

I recall one day walking into the room of a patient, a lovely woman that I cared about, and she was dealing with a serious illness and several associated complications. I approached her room thinking about how I was going to help her and worrying about her treatment. When I entered her room she asked, "What's wrong?"

"Why are you asking me that?" I responded.

"Your face and forehead are all wrinkled."

"I am thinking about how to help you."

"Think in the hallway, then," she said. "I need you to smile when you come in here." She was right. I needed an attitude adjustment to be a better physician for her, and it was an adjustment I happily made. The best doctors learn from the critiques and coaching supplied by their patients, nurses, and families. I learned from all of these people that when I lightened up, encouraged laughter in others, and practiced it myself, everybody benefited.

One good example of laughter changing a tense situation is illustrated by an anxious woman who was afraid to have surgery. I had spent almost an hour trying to calm her down in the hallway outside the operating room, until finally realizing that nothing I said was help-ing her. So we wheeled her into the OR, and in her panic she blurted out, "Thank God all these wonderful people are going to be taking care of me."

I knew if I agreed with her it wouldn't help. So, loudly enough for everyone to hear, I said, "I know these people. I have worked with them for years, and they are not wonderful people." There were two seconds of bewildered looks, and then she and everyone in the room burst out laughing; we all became family and she did beautifully.

Another experience that convinced me about the value of humor occurred when my wife and I were out lecturing. Bobbie used to do a stand-up comedy act delivering one-liners as part of the presenta-tion. This was a sort of intermission that gave people a break from the lecture. Instead of listening to more of my stories about exceptional-patient behavior, they got a chance to *experience* some of our group therapy methods.

When I introduced Bobbie, I would say, "Here's my wife, Bob-bie; she's like a female Henny Youngman, and we have had thirty-eight wonderful years of married life." The women would all smile at me until I concluded with, "and thirty-eight out of fifty-six isn't too bad." Then their expressions would change, and moments later the first laughter would erupt.

Usually when Bobbie did her routine, I would take her seat in the audience and enjoy the show. One time, however, there was a place for me to sit at the back of the stage, so I was able to observe the audience. The change in their physical appearance after laughing for fifteen to twenty minutes was striking and made me a firm believer in the benefits of humor. They looked so much healthier! Their eyes shone, and their postures were open and relaxed. Bobbie often ended her routine with the statement "He who laughs, lasts." And her final piece of advice was: Laughter is contagious, so be a carrier.

After witnessing the remarkable change in that audience, I always made it a point to discuss the benefits of laughter before Bobbie did her routine, so people would be aware of how they were changed physically by the experience. And you know what? Bobbie always received more thank-yous at the end of the evening than I did.

I recommend that you use spontaneous laughter and maintain a childlike sense of humor throughout your day. When I talk about childlike humor, it's about seeing the world through a child's eyes. For example, if you see a sign that says, WET FLOOR, go ahead and do it. When the instructions at the front desk say, "Sign In Upon Entering," sign the register using those words: *In Upon Entering*. This can lead to a long wait, but it's fun. When a form says, "Print Your Name," print: "YOUR NAME" in bold letters. When the sign says, NOBODY ALLOWED HERE, go in, and when they shout at you to get out of there, tell them, "I'm a nobody. I can go in." Most of the time the guards let you go, thinking if you're that stupid, you're no danger. Once when I did that, a guard stepped in front of me and said, "I'm making you a Somebody. You have to leave now." The guard's inner child had appeared, and so I gave him a hug.

When a radio interviewer asked me how I managed to be happy during these difficult and challenging times, I told her, "I have learned that you must always finish everything you begin. So before I leave home in the morning, the first thing I do is finish all the red and white wine, the kahlua, Prozac, and Valium in the house. By the time I go out the door, I feel really happy." There was a pause before she started to giggle. She got it — one of the best ways to be happy, especially when everything is collapsing around you, is just to laugh.

In *Anatomy of an Illness as Perceived by the Patient*, Norman Cousins wrote a fascinating account of his self-induced healing-by-laughter from a diagnosed condition, ankylosing spondylitis. When his doctor gave him a one-in-five-hundred chance of recovery, Cousins checked himself into a hotel, watched *Candid Camera* tapes, and laughed, day after day.[1] Choosing to use humor as his medicine, rather than react to his fear and do nothing, is the sign of an optimist — a survivor.

The opposite of optimism (a sign of happiness) is negativity (a lack of hope and the unawareness of potential). Negativity is an attitude that stems from fear: "Oh no, this is going to happen; that's going to happen." How can you be happy when you're afraid, when the first thought in your mind is the worst-case scenario?

Fear is meant to help you save your life. If you are walking in the woods and you see a snake that might be poisonous, then fear is an appropriate reaction. You'll jump back instinctively. I had that happen the other day while riding my bike through the woods. I thought I saw something that looked like a coyote or a wolf, and I swerved the bike without even thinking. Then I realized it was only a branch with a shadow, but it looked just like an animal ready to attack. What amazed me was that I had already changed the direction of my bike before my brain had had time to say, "It's okay, it's just a shadow."

Fear is appropriate when a snarling dog lunges at you with teeth bared. Your heart rate increases and, with a rush of adrenaline, you find the strength to climb a tree that previously you couldn't climb. But if you live in a constant state of fear, it is as if you are walking in the woods where everything around you is a poisonous snake or a rabid dog. Your body is constantly being pumped with stress chemicals that wear you down. It cannot repair itself when it's putting all that energy into the fight-or-flight response, the automatic reaction of self-preservation. When you live in constant or chronic fear, your immune system becomes weakened as levels of stress hormones go up, causing increased blood sugar and inflammation of the circulatory system.

Patients sometimes reveal hidden fears in their drawings about family situations, their disease, or their treatment. These fears will not be expressed verbally during a visit to the doctor, so he can do nothing to help the patient through them. If you can get the patient to talk about this fear via their drawing, and turn it around so that they can see the humorous side of their situation and laugh about it, the laughter will beneficially affect their treatment and recovery outcome. (See my commentary on fig. 47 in chapter 6.)

If you live with thoughts of love and engage in daily laughter, the opposite of what you worried about happens. It is nearly impossible to live in fear when you laugh, and when you laugh every day your outlook changes. How can this be? You come to realize that *you* control two things: your thoughts and behaviors. Happiness is not a place you arrive at or an award you receive; it is something you practice, and in the practicing you *become* happy as a result of your attitude, thoughts, and behavior.

Think of yourself as an actor; rehearse until you are happy with your performance. Even when acting, an actor's body chemistry is altered by the emotions related to the role she is playing, whether it is a comedy or tragedy.

Ingrid Bergman told a funny story about working with Alfred Hitchcock. She was supposed to play an emotional scene in the film, and each time she tried she couldn't feel the part. Confessing to Hitchcock that she didn't think she could give that kind of emotion, the straight-faced director looked at the actress and said, "Ingrid, *fake* it."[2]

This does not mean you should pretend you aren't sad when, say, your dog dies. Negative emotions as reactions to life challenges are normal, but when you use them to give yourself permission to hang on to fear or to wallow in sad, dark thoughts, they become destructive. It is normal to grieve over the dog, or to cry when your knee is scraped after skidding off your bike, but once the flow of tears has run its course, find something funny about the situation and start laughing. Roll in it; love it; let tears of laughter wash the negative emotions away and the healing process begins.

Scientists have studied the effects of laughter on the body and identified a number of physiological benefits. Laughter increases activity in the immune system, giving "good" killer cells a boost, especially in their ability to target viruses, some tumors, and cancer cells. Measurements of immune system components show a lingering beneficial effect from laughter that lasts *into the next day*. Laughter appears to fight infection and abrasion or chemical insults to the upper tract of the respiratory system. Laughter is a natural muscle-relaxant; at the same time, it provides a good cardiac and diaphragm workout, improving the body's capacity to use oxygen. This makes it an ideal activity for those whose ability to exercise is limited. Laughter also improves mood and decreases patients' perception or awareness of pain. As in the case of appropriate exercise, there are no negative side effects to laughter.

Many years ago I fell off our roof when the top rung of a ladder I was climbing broke. When I told this story to an audience, I said, "I must have an angel, because I landed on my feet. Considering the angle of the ladder, landing on my feet seemed impossible." At the end of my talk, a man came up to me and said, "You do have an angel, and I know his name."

"How do you know?" I asked.

"What did you say when the ladder broke?"

"Oh, shit."

"That's your angel's name," he said.

I laughed, not realizing at the time the gift he gave me. Now, whenever I get into a difficult situation and yell out, "Oh, shit," I start laughing because I know help is on the way. Feel free to make use of my guardian angel whenever you are in need. That man from the audience has helped me get through many things, including the time I hit a sheet of ice while on my bike and flew into the air, only to yell, "Oh, shit!" When I hit the ground laughing, I was completely relaxed and, consequently, sustained no injuries.

Laughter yoga is a form of exercise that incorporates breathing and laughter without the use of jokes or comedy movies. It is based on the premise that the body does not recognize the difference between spontaneous and forced laughter, and that the beneficial effects are the same. Fifteen minutes of belly laughter is reported to be the minimum time required to get the best physiological results. Natural laughter usually lasts for a few seconds, but laughter yoga exercises keep the laughter flowing for as long as the person wishes.

Laughter yoga is similar to the Zen Buddhism practice of forced laughter. Some participants may find it awkward at first, but the faked laughter soon becomes genuine, and the phrase "Fake it till you make it" could easily be applied to laughter yoga. I have done these exercises and found it very hard to stop laughing even when there was no reason to laugh.

DOCTOR'S R_x

Try this in front of the mirror or while facing a friend: Raise your eyebrows, take a deep breath, and chant the meditation sound *Ohm* for three seconds. Then relax your eyebrows, smile, and make as many *hee, hee, hee* sounds as you can until you have expelled all of your breath. While faking the laughter, make sure to keep a big smile on your face, even if it feels like a grimace. Take another deep breath, raise your eyebrows, and chant *Ohm* for three seconds. Then relax your eyebrows, smile, and chant *Ha, ha, ha* until your breath is used up.

Do this several times, switching between sounds and allowing any natural laughter that bubbles up to take over and replace the fake laughter. Even if natural laughter doesn't happen, do the exercise for fifteen minutes. Notice how you feel when you're finished.

Senior centers and nursing homes that facilitate laughter classes have reported that residents enjoy the sessions and ask for more. They forget their aches and pains, and people report a lift in their overall mood during and after the sessions and up to twenty-four hours later.

THE LAST LAUGH

I suggest that when you are ready to die, have your family tell stories about your life as they sit with you. My father literally died laughing as my mother told wonderful stories about their early relationship. Dad was tired of his body and had told Mom, "I need to get out of here." She was able to let go of him and knew he was going to die that day. We were called to come. I went out to exercise before we left home, and I heard a voice ask, "How did your parents meet?" I answered that I didn't know, and the voice said, "Then ask your mother when you get to the hospital."

Several hours later, when we walked into Dad's hospital room, the inner voice reminded me to ask the question, so I said, "How did you two meet?"

Mom described how she was on a vacation and had been sitting on the beach with girls she didn't know, girls who, she later learned, had a very bad reputation. Some boys came walking down the beach, and they flipped coins to see who would get which girl. Then she told us, "Your father lost and got me."

On their second date he took her rowing, and as he was helping her into the boat, the man who owned it yelled out, "Hey, you have to pay before you get in the boat."

"Your dad let go of me and the boat," Mom said, "and I fell into the water. Things got even worse after that...," and everyone in the room was laughing. Dad was in a coma by then, but I knew he could still hear us, and at some level he was joining in the laughter. He looked so good that I thought he was going to postpone dying, but as soon as the last grandchild arrived he departed his body, leaving everyone with a feeling of wholeness and no fear of death.

I ask seniors to tell me how they can die laughing. Their answers relate to two accomplishments. One is their having completed what we are all here to do, which is to serve the world in our unique way rather than in a way determined by others. When people spend their lives doing what they love, laughter comes much easier at the end. The second accomplishment is their collection of stories about times in their life that may have been difficult, maddening, or embarrassing when they happened, but which elicit hoots of laughter now. Sometimes these stories come from their adult kids saying, "Dad, I was so embarrassed when you did that; I was trying to pretend you were some other kid's father," and they get to enjoy a hilarious family moment once again.

So remember, don't be afraid to embarrass your family and give them material to use when you are ready to die — and die laughing at their stories. Like the time we couldn't find one of our rescued exotic pets. I decided to call the police, in case anyone reported seeing it. Imagine calling the police to say you couldn't find your kinkajou: "Your what?" "Yes, my kinkajou. He went missing." When the kids heard me call the police the first time, they thought it was embarrassing enough, but when I called the next time, they heard me saying that I had found my kinkajou in the rafters of the house by walking around up there with a banana until he stuck his head out.

Name your dog Sex and your cats Hope and Miracle, as I have. See what happens when you run around the yard chasing Sex and shout to your wife that you don't have Miracle and can't get Sex, but at least you've got Hope. You'll embarrass your kids with your childlike humor, but they will appreciate it later in life.

Our children come home and say, "Thanks, Dad." When I ask why, they say they did something crazy at work or at school, and instead of people around them complaining or criticizing, those people say to each other, "Well, you know who his father is."

Be a collector of funny events that happen, and make them into unforgettable memories by sharing them and writing them down. I often ask for Chinese food when I go to pick up my takeout order at Ernie's Pizzeria. Pat, the owner, knows me and loves that I am nuts, but new waitresses don't know what to do with me, as they try to explain I'm in the wrong restaurant. One night I walked in and asked for my Chinese food, and the waitress put out three containers of Chinese food; the whole restaurant burst into laughter. My behavior also kept our five kids from eating out with me and saved me a lot of money.

Terry Bruce wrote to me saying that sharing funny stories about her children helped to heal a difficult relationship with her mother.

Sometimes Mum drives me crazy, and I have a tendency to snap at her, which always leaves me feeling worse because we only get to visit each other every couple of years. One day I was already tired when she called, and I knew this could be a bad day to talk. But Mum started reminiscing about funny things my kids had done on her last trip over here, so I sat and listened.

She reminded me about the day we'd all gone blackberry picking. When we got back to the house, I poured all the berries into a bowl. My three-year-old daughter had picked two blackberries out of the bowl and put them into her mouth. "Izzy, don't eat any more of those," I said, "or there won't be enough for dessert." With a look of pure innocence on her face, Izzy replied, "I wasn't eating them, Mummy. I was rinsing them." Then she took the berries out of her mouth and placed them back in the bowl.

Mum and I laughed, and that story reminded me of things that my other children, Farley, Raffy, and Jesse, had done. Many were precious moments that Mum had missed seeing, but now as I shared them in graphic detail we were laughing again. By the time we hung up, I felt really close to her, as if she'd been here. And rather than driving each other crazy, we thoroughly enjoyed our call. That powerful sense of family and belonging gave me a boost for the rest of the day. All the things that I had been stressing about before suddenly seemed insignificant.

The world is filled with pain. The world is also a human comedy if we choose to see it that way. Yes, it is a tragic comedy at times, but you can still be a healer and spread joy through humor and laughter. Why do you think Shakespeare's comedies are still so appealing more than four hundred years after he wrote them? It's because people love to laugh. Something deep inside us knows it is good for us. After a funeral, go to the wake and watch how quickly people begin to share funny stories. Something inside them is saying it's time to heal a little. So, have a laugh; heal the wounds of grief, and don't put out your loved one's celestial candle with your tears.

My friend Diane was having a family reunion with her sister and two brothers, and they fell into fits of laughter over stories of their stepmother's thriftiness. "I couldn't believe it that time I went to visit Mom and Dad," Diane shared with her siblings, "and when I got up to go and use the bathroom, Mom said, 'Don't use the good toilet paper, dear. I save that for guests.'"

Her brother Bruce added, "Yeah, and after Dad died she announced she had something to give us. I was hoping it might be an envelope with a check in it or maybe something that had belonged to Dad, like his war medals. I nearly fell over when she reached into her purse and pulled out four ziplock freezer bags filled with ashes. 'Here's your dad,' she said and gave him back to us."

"Do you remember what you did?" asked Diane. "You held up your bag and asked Mom, 'Which end of Dad did I get?'"

The ensuing laughter renewed family bonds and helped to heal old resentments. It is hard to hold a grudge when the root of the resentment produces such colorful stories to inspire hilarious fits of laughter.

BE INFECTIOUS

Several years ago my wife came home from shopping and went into the bathroom. I went out to the car, brought in all the groceries and put them away. When she returned to the kitchen, I was expecting a big thank-you and much praise for what I had done. Instead she said, "You don't put tomatoes in the refrigerator." That hurt my feelings. No thank-you — just criticism. So I wrote a poem titled "Divorce."

> Tomatoes don't belong in the refrigerator
> I did it again
> my wife may never forgive me
> our marriage is on the rocks
> I snore, put tomatoes in the fridge
> and I walk and eat too fast
> the divorce lawyer doesn't know how

to help us reach a valid settlement
for my cruelty
he suggests we try to work it out
to give love a chance
and don't put tomatoes in the fridge
I read his settlement to my wife
she laughs
I love her when she laughs
and forget the difficult times
we fire the lawyer
and take the tomatoes out of the fridge[3]

When I read this to Bobbie she laughed, and, just as the poem says, I love her when she laughs. I'll also share a few things Bobbie warns people to look out for. She calls them "Bobbie's Warning Signs":

- You call your wife to say you'd like to have dinner out, and she leaves a sandwich on the front porch.
- You put your bra on backwards and it fits better.
- You call suicide prevention, and they put you on hold.
- You call the missing person's bureau, and they tell you to get lost.
- The fortune-teller offers you a refund.
- You come home from the beauty parlor and your dog growls and won't let you in the house.
- You open a fortune cookie and find a summons.
- The bird sitting outside your window is a vulture.

And here's some wise marriage advice from my wife:

- Never go to bed mad. Stay up and fight.
- Never argue with a woman when she is tired or rested.

- Next time your hubby is angry say, "You are so handsome when you are angry."

Love her? You bet I love her.

For some people, laughter comes easy; for others, it takes practice, often owing to childhood experiences where laughter was not encouraged. Artists must practice their skill in order to explore, learn, and grow in the mastery of their craft, whether they are painting, writing, or doing any other form of creative expression. The key word here is expression. So I recommend that you practice the expression of giggles and guffaws; become an artist, and fill your palette with laughter. Remember it's not healthy to be serious and normal. Trying to be normal is only for those who feel inadequate. So be an infectious carrier. Spread joy and healing, and keep the artist within you alive.

Chapter 9

FAKE IT TILL YOU MAKE IT

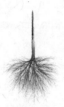

Keep your face to the sunshine, and you cannot see the shadow.

— HELEN KELLER

When we consider the relationship between parenting and health, we often do so only within the context of children's health and forget about the importance of parents' health. But parental health and parental love — for self and for one's children — are the most significant public health factors on the planet.

As the father of five children, including twins, all of them born within a period of seven years, I know the role that exhaustion played in my wife's health and mine. When the children were young, we slept only a few hours each night as we cared for the kids, prepared formula, cleaned diapers, played with them, and watched over them. We were acting out of love, but the fatigue had its effect on our immune systems and stress hormone levels. The result was that I ended up in the hospital with a severe staphylococcal infection, and my wife developed multiple sclerosis.

One of the things all parents should do is take time to get away and restore themselves. There is no need to feel guilty over occasionally leaving your children and caring for yourself, giving yourself the opportunity to live an authentic life rather than a role. Once we learned our lesson about taking better care of ourselves, at the beginning of each year Bobbie would get the calendar out and determine how many days we could be caring parents before it took a toll on our health. Then she'd reserve several days every few months, so that she and I could go off together while friends or family would take our place and share their time and affection with our children.

Everyone benefited from the separation. Through our neighbors, friends, and my patients, our children found a new set of experienced parents and grandparents who were willing and ready to listen to their problems and love them, and my wife and I had a chance to restore ourselves and relate to things other than diapers, schedules, and meals. It also gave our kids a chance to play games with adults who didn't know all their devious techniques for outsmarting parents.

I have had many patients who developed a dependence on food, drugs, alcohol, or other addictive behaviors, and what I learned from them was that this was their response to a childhood in which they experienced indifference, rejection, or abuse — the opposite of love — from their parents. They sought to reward themselves in order to feel better, but these choices were self-destructive for they were only temporary fixes. People who choose a path of self-destruction don't live that way because of a lack of information. What they lack is inspiration and a sense of self-worth.

A study that followed a group of Harvard students revealed that, of the students who felt their parents did not love them, by midlife almost 100 percent had suffered a major illness. In comparison, among those who felt loved, only 25 percent developed a major illness during the same period.

As children develop, they require, at very specific times, certain kinds of messages from one or both parents that will make the children feel loved and secure. Most people probably don't realize that until a child reaches the age of six, his or her brainwave pattern is similar to that of a hypnotized individual. By the time children become capable of evaluating their parents' words, they have a real struggle on their hands to free themselves from the negative messages most parents deliver. When those messages are destructive, it's really difficult to get beyond them.

To quote one of my patients: "My mother's words were eating away at me and maybe even gave me cancer." This woman's mother had constantly belittled her accomplishments and dressed her only in dark colors so she would not be noticed by others. She had to develop a life-threatening illness before she could go out and buy a red dress, begin a new life, and become her authentic self.

When parents impose behavior patterns, career choices, and more, what they are often doing is literally taking their child's life away. The sweet identical twin sister who pleases Mom, Dad, and the family, but internalizes anger, is far more likely to develop breast cancer later in life than her little devil of a sister who is always doing her own thing.

Parenting problems can be revealed in the drawings made by children. For example, a child might draw a family picture and give her mother a facial expression that makes her look as if she's angry and using verbal aggression, and draw her father with his hands in his pockets and facing away from the mother, showing his emotional withdrawal. She might draw her own facial expression as looking sad or frightened. When this drawing is brought to the parents' attention, they are more easily motivated to get help. Rather than hearing the therapist's interpretation, which makes them feel they are bad parents, they see what their child says with pictures, what she is going through; this tells them what they need to hear.

Family counseling, classes in parenting and anger control, and workshops in communication skills are often the key to helping the family work as a unit. Not only will this ease the child's psychological distress, but it will also play a big part in healing the child's physical disease and create for her a healthier mind and body for the rest of her life.

We must recognize the importance of listening to one another and verbalizing our love. Be sure to give your children love even when you don't like what they are doing. Do not attack them with words like: "There's something wrong with you." Instead use words that say, "I love you, but what you are doing is unsafe and unhealthy, so please stop." Let them know you do not like their behavior while, at the same time, you reassure them that you love them. The teen years can be the most challenging for kids, especially when their parents have not developed an open channel of loving communication. When the kids need guidance and support, they don't feel they can go to the parents with their problems or ask them for help. In one study, 70 percent of high school students said they had considered suicide. These kids have no idea how to eliminate what is killing them, so they consider killing themselves.

Remember that the opposite of love is not hate but indifference, rejection, or abuse. Why do I think children become bullies? When they receive mottoes to die by from the authority figures in their lives and witness other negative behaviors in an unloving environment, they will act out in ways that are destructive to themselves and others, using bullying tactics, aggression, and violence. These children do not interpret aggression the same way we do, because children who develop in a violent, unloving environment have a nervous system that is far less sensitive to physical aggression, noise, and other sensory stimuli. Parts of their brains literally shut down. Studies have shown that neglect, trauma, and abuse in childhood have a physical impact on the central nervous system — the brain, spinal cord, and nerves — leaving some structures and pathways underdeveloped and other structures and pathways overdeveloped.[1]

Children may deliberately act out. The troublemaker gets attention; even if it is negative attention, it feels better than rejection. Aggression is a normal feeling, but in order to get attention, and sometimes revenge, the unloved and rejected child will turn healthy aggression into violence and destruction rather than engage in sports, work, and hobbies.

Just as fire can either heat or destroy your home, so the energy within children can be directed to healthy endeavors. Children can rebel in healthy ways and not by bullying. When their energy is directed into something positive, such as engaging with the arts, sports, hobbies, or volunteering, the world becomes a better place, and no one is threatened by that energy. We need to provide such outlets and help children search for what fulfills their needs in a healthy way.

As a boy, I became jealous of a neighbor's toy; I acted like a bully and broke it. When my father came home and learned what I had done, he said nothing to me about it; but the following day he came home with the same toy. He didn't tell me what to do with it. He just handed it to me and walked away. My father's action spoke more to me than any words of chastisement would. He did the right thing as the responsible adult by replacing the broken toy, but he left me with the decision of whether to keep it or give it to my neighbor. His action told me that he loved me, trusted me, and wanted me to do the right thing. Whether I did that or not was my decision. My father knew that what he was putting me through was worse than physical punishment. And yes, I went over and gave it to my neighbor.

We need to convey a reverence for life to children. We can do this by teaching them how to be responsible for the life and comfort of some living thing, be it a plant, pet, or another human being, and give them the opportunity to do so with appropriate supervision. When you care for and about what you live with, you respect the world and its inhabitants.

My wife and I filled our home and yard with rescued animals. We broke every zoning law, but no one, including the police, ever reported us, because they knew we were caring for all these creatures. Our children even carried insects out of the house because they respected them as living things. When the children reached the age of rebellion, instead of directing their energy against people, they focused it on improving the status quo and creating a better world. When they needed love and attention, they asked for it or did crazy things, but they never acted in a destructive way toward anyone or anything.

As an example, one son would tell us the grandparents had called and wanted him to visit them. So I would put him on a bus to go see them. As an adult he confessed they never called; he just needed to get away and get some loving. He was the one who, when Bobbie and I were away, got his siblings to tell the couple staying with them that he had left early for school. But he didn't go to school; he was sitting in the cedar closet all day reading books. He knew how to get attention and also how to care for himself without hurting anyone.

Anger needs to be expressed appropriately, not repressed. When children are angry, ask them why. Listen to them and help them find a safe way to deal with the cause of their anger, as well as a way to release and externalize their feelings. When hospital staff members continually barged into his room for insignificant reasons, a dying teenager used a water gun to let people know he wanted privacy. His anger hurt no one and taught many nurses and doctors to respect his needs as a human being living under difficult circumstances, rather than think of him merely as a hospital patient who needed scheduled management. The boy's water gun became a gift for other children to use after he died. As a parent what do you do if your hospitalized child is being treated like a disease rather than a person? Take along a Siegel Kit, as I mentioned in chapter 6 (see page 95).

And what do you do if your child is being picked on by a bully at school or in the neighborhood? It is appropriate for your child to be angry when not treated with respect, but to respond to violence with violence only aggravates the situation. I would make the authorities at school or in your neighborhood aware of what is happening, but I would also kill with kindness and torment with tenderness. Be creative in your approach. I have seen love dissolve a bad situation even when someone's life was being threatened.

Tell your child to invite the bully over to your house for some fun and games. Or go someplace together, such as an amusement park, and enjoy a good meal. Call the bully's parents and chat with them about their child's behavior. If you were to learn the bully's mom had been diagnosed with cancer, or that the parents are alcoholics, you would find it easier to understand and forgive the bully, and your child would learn more about being a genuine friend. If you try it and it doesn't work, then eliminate the relationship.

Once I was speaking in a classroom at a school in a dangerous neighborhood, and just before my lecture four boys came in and took the front-row seats. This struck me as odd because students don't often choose to sit right in front of the teacher. I later learned that these four boys were the school gang leader and his bodyguards, and those were their seats in every classroom. I asked a question, and the gang leader raised his hand to answer. When he was done, I told him that was not the right answer and I went on to explain why. The principal revealed afterward that the boy hadn't spoken in a class in four years. He expressed his concern: now that I had told the gang leader he was wrong, what was he going to do to the school? I told the principal not to worry. The boy knew I was there only because I cared about him and the other students, and he was having a good time. There was no trouble afterward. By talking respectfully and honestly with those kids, and by sharing a little bit of wisdom and a lot of laughter, I had planted a seed of love.

Through our persistent love, even when we do not like what the bullies are doing, we can reparent them and help them to rebel against the elements of our society that need to change. When we do this, the bullies come to realize they are worth loving and begin to care about themselves and others. I have seen this with children, patients, and other people I have developed relationships with through my work.

I love to bring senior citizens and students together, because everyone needs a loving grandparent who is filled with the wisdom of a lifetime. When you do this, you establish guidance: god-u-and-i-dance. Even people in nursing homes are valuable teachers when they get the opportunity to be with students. Older people often teach children that troubles can be instances of redirection from which something good will come.

If I had to summarize how to raise a healthy child, I'd suggest you get a puppy, go to a veterinarian, and ask how to raise your puppy. Then go home and do the same thing with your child. To quote some vets I know: "Consistency, respect, affection, discipline, love, and exercise." The acronym for this is CRADLE, and it sounds good to me.

For more details on this topic, read my book *Love, Magic & Mudpies* about how to raise children who feel loved, who practice kindness, and who make a positive difference in the world. All too often children grow into adulthood without such help, and they are left to cope with the physical, emotional, and mental consequences of bad parenting.

REPARENTING

If something was going on in your family during the formative years in your life, something that interfered with your getting loving, positive messages from the important adults in your life, then you need to *reparent* yourself. It is actually damaging you when you listen to the voices of your past telling you that in some way you are not good enough. The way to get out of the negative trance and change your self-image is by actively and intentionally leaving those old recordings and unhappy experiences behind. By the time we are adults, it's not about blaming our parents. It's about becoming empowered and making our own choices.

I recommend that you start by getting to know yourself as a little child. In your mind, separate the person you are today from the child you were, and get ready to love that divine child as if he or she exists right here, right now, because that child does exist — within you. No matter how crazy you think this idea sounds, try it anyway. Fake it till you make it.

Use this method: Find photographs of yourself as a child and place them where you spend your time so you will see them daily. I call them shrines. Fall in love with that child. Talk to her or him. Tell her that she is safe and loved and will grow to be strong. Tell him how wonderful it is that he was born, and that he is valuable and has a purpose in your life.

Carry the image of that child in your mind and heart throughout the day, and every time you feel disturbed, anxious, or afraid, imagine that it is the child who is having those feelings. Ask yourself, what would I do to comfort this kid? Then do it for yourself. Just as hunger leads you to seek nourishment, use these feelings to direct you into nourishing your life in the ways it needs to be nourished.

On a daily basis, once you have reparented the child inside yourself, extend that loving care to your outer adult self. If you had a son or daughter who was bullied day after day by a teacher whose comments were damaging your child's self-esteem, wouldn't you go to the teacher and insist that she treat your child with kindness and respect? If the teacher didn't change her behavior, wouldn't you have your child transferred to another class where the teacher encouraged the children and made learning an enjoyable experience? If another class wasn't made available, wouldn't you remove your child from that school?

Do the same for yourself now. Talk to your unfair manager at work or to anyone who treats you badly. Tell him you love him, but you don't like how he is treating you, and that you expect to be treated with kindness and respect. If he doesn't change his behavior, you can always walk away from that job or relationship. Put yourself in situations where you will not be damaged by the toxic behaviors of others. Sometimes you can't change your life, but you can change your attitude. When your health is threatened, changing your life by walking away is best; but if you can't, developing a positive change in attitude can do wonders. When you choose happiness, it affects everyone around you.

While you're at it, talk to the critic in your head. When you make a mistake, does the voice in your head accuse you of being stupid, worthless, or otherwise not good enough? If you saw a child make a mistake, I hope you would say, "It's okay; everybody makes mistakes. Mistakes are an important part of learning." I know of a golf instructor who tells her students not to judge the results of a swing with the mental comment "Wow, that was great," or "Oh no, that was awful." She tells her students to practice saying, "That was *interesting*." This gives the mind permission to learn from each swing without setting up an expectation or demand, on the one hand, or a sense of failure, on the other. Both of these mind-sets work against the brain's learning mechanisms.

So when you make a mistake, stop yelling at yourself. Be as kind and gentle with yourself as you would be with a child. Use mistakes as a tool, not as a humiliating instance of failure. When we learn how not to do something, next time we can do it differently. Laugh at yourself, forgive yourself, and move on. You have the potential.

TWELVE-STEP PROGRAMS

People were not designed to live life alone. We are tribal by nature and form communities for biological and psychosocial survival. People who join groups of individuals who face challenges similar to their own often turn their lives around, especially when they meet in an atmosphere of nonjudgment and anonymity. When the "natives" who have lived the experience come together, they can truly help one another. The "tourists," on the other hand, do not understand what the natives are experiencing and will make suggestions and comments or prescribe things that are of no help.

Sharing our experience allows us to help each other through the journey of life and its difficulties. We become potential teachers the minute we face the mountain that sits before us. In the ECaP groups I facilitate, bonds formed by patients often last for years, and people feel like they're family. Often the families people adopt are healthier and less judgmental than the ones they were born into.

Alcoholics Anonymous was the first twelve-step program of fellowship, and it was developed by two men who could not stop drinking despite trying absolutely everything in their power to quit. From its humble origin in 1935 to now, AA has grown to over two million active members in recovery across the world.[2] Other twelve-step groups have evolved from the original: Al-Anon and Alateen are for families of alcoholics, ACA is for the adult children of alcoholics, OA is for overeaters, GA is for gamblers, and so on. Wikipedia lists more than thirty such programs based on the original Twelve Steps and Twelve Traditions of Alcoholics Anonymous.

If your life seems to be repeating the same negative patterns and is spiraling out of control, look up the twelve-step meetings in your area. Go to a meeting and listen. You'll be surprised to find people whose stories have similarities to yours, and you will experience relief when you discover a place where you feel you belong.

Years ago I told cancer patients who had no local support groups to go to an AA meeting and lie about why they were there. Some AA members felt I was doing the wrong thing, but the principles and practices of AA have proven to be sound, and these people needed help. If a theme repeats itself as an aid to recovery, then be assured it must work — or you wouldn't find it in the Bible, in Buddha's teachings, or at a support group meeting.

LIVING IN THE MOMENT

Slow down and feel your feelings. Living mindfully and in the moment requires that you become aware of your feelings and accept them as your own creation. Don't hide from your feelings by keeping busy, distracting yourself, or by self-medicating to numb yourself. We cannot heal what we don't feel.

After I expressed my anger over family problems that I couldn't fix, and all the diseases I couldn't cure, my close friend Elisabeth Kübler-Ross said quietly to me during one of her workshops: "You have needs, too." Those words have stayed with me, and I share them with you now as an important truth to remember.

One place where we store our feelings is in our hearts. Even transplanted hearts hold feelings and carry messages from the donor's life. When evaluating options and choices or making decisions, let your heart become the compass point. One woman shared her father's advice with me. Before he died, Fred Croker advised his daughter to "follow your heart and use your mind to navigate the heart-chosen path."

Let your feelings be the guide to what inspires you. Let them not only fill your lungs with inspiration but also fill your every activity with life and the joy that comes from having creative choices. Accept that the way you felt about something in the past may not be the way you feel about it today. Allow yourself to know and honor the person you are today and not hang on to something that no longer serves you. By doing so, you become a cocreator of your life. I like to remember what my mother always said when I had a decision to make: "Do what makes you happy." When things didn't go as I had planned, she reminded me: "God is redirecting you. Something good will come of this."

Practice paying attention to the moment rather than the past or the future. Focus on your breath. If you're breathing, things are looking good. Stay out of other people's thoughts; their thoughts and attitudes are not your business, not even what they think about you. Your job is to be the best you can be in this moment, dealing with whatever is directly in front of you, one small step at a time. And when you need help, ask for it. As one of my favorite songs by Tom Hunter says, "Tonight I'd like you to rock me to sleep."[3]

When you live in the moment, you begin to realize that a perfect world would be meaningless, giving you no choices or possibilities for growth.

HONOR THYSELF

Find your authentic life and do not live a role. Don't be the Wage Earner or the Momma, because if you believe the role is who you are, you lose the meaning of your life when you can no longer work or the kids grow up and leave home. There is a story about a man who stood at the gates of heaven, asking to come in. "Tell me who you are," God said. The man thought about his wife and family and all the people he had worked hard to please. He thought about his important job, impressive house, and fancy car. He thought about the bills piling up on his desk and the cruise vacation he and his wife had been planning. All these thoughts circled around him, and no matter how hard he tried, he could remember only the roles he played. "I don't know who I am," he admitted.

"Then you are not ready to enter," God replied and sent the man back to his body. When the man recovered from his heart attack, he made a pledge to find his authentic self.

Over the next few years, the man learned that the heart speaks in whispers, which meant the man had to slow down at least once a day, be still, and listen. He stopped trying to impress others and worked instead on the things he loved doing. He took time to listen to people without interrupting or rushing them, and he valued the growth in his relationships. The more he focused on the here and now, the more he seemed to accomplish. He was able to be of service to people in many small ways, and when the small things added up, they made a big difference in the world around him.

As time went by, he realized he felt good about himself, and the new behaviors that had once taken concentrated effort were now ingrained habits. Life and death placed no fearful images in front of him but were instead mirrors that reflected love and integrity. Several more years passed before the man approached the gates of heaven for the second time.

"Tell me who you are," God said.

"I am Wholeness. I am your divine child. I am you," said the man.

"Welcome home, my child," said God, and the man was embraced by a light more brilliant than the sun.

I knew a teenager who, as he lay dying, said, "Tell God his replacement is here." He was admitted immediately.

I am reminded of a patient of mine who was diagnosed with agoraphobia. When this woman, who had been unable to leave her house for years, learned that she had only two months to live, she saw the light and asked herself, "What is the point of being afraid?" From a person living with a crippling condition that stopped her from going out in the rain, she changed into a woman who took up white-water rafting! It scared the wits out of her kids, but it also led to her surviving cancer. And a letter I received from another woman with a similar prognosis ended with, "And I didn't die, and now I am so busy I'm killing myself."

You *do* have control of your thoughts and actions, so take control — it is your right. Rehearse being the person you want to be, and each day *act* like you are already that person. If you are afraid, imagine loving arms around you before you fall asleep, so that when you awaken you will immediately think of that warm, comforting thought to push away the fear. Or if you need a role model when in doubt, ask yourself, "What would Lassie do" (WWLD)?

JOURNALING

In a study of a group of people who suffered from asthma, individuals were told to keep a journal of their feelings about their experiences for a month, while the control group was told to simply list what they did each day. After a month, those who wrote about their feelings and experiences proved to have better health and suffered fewer asthma attacks than the people who only listed what they did every day.

The other day I was looking through some of my papers while searching for something, and I found my journals from twenty-five to thirty-five years ago. As a doctor, I had begun to make notes during the day about things that affected me, and then at home in the evening I would write about them in my journal. Soon after I started this practice, I found that when I tried to write about what had happened during the day, I couldn't remember what my notes referred to. Imagine writing "child in emergency room" and twelve hours later asking myself,

"What was that about?" I realized then that, whatever the pain was, it was in me and I couldn't deal with it; so I was burying it and storing it within my body. The haunting words *Someday the body will present its bill* came to mind, and I began to write whole paragraphs in my notes so I would remember what I needed to deal with in my journal.

Once, when I forgot to hide my journal, my wife found it and read it. Bobbie said, "Bernie, there's nothing funny in here." I said, "What are you talking about? My life isn't funny." She then reminded me of crazy things that had happened in the hospital and that had had the whole family laughing when I shared the story. These stories had never made it into my journal. Bobbie's comment refocused me so that I started looking at the nice things that happened as well: you get a hug; you get a little love; you get a little laughter. "Put that in your journal, too," she said, and I did.

Writing a journal keeps you aware and lets your unconscious know you're willing to deal with whatever turmoil is inside you. We all need to be heard by someone who cares. In order for our inner voice to speak to us, we have to find a way to listen to it. Writing gives us the means to listen. I've often referred to Helen Keller's observation that "deafness is a much worse misfortune [than blindness]." Survival behavior requires you to know what is in your heart, reveal the unconscious, and feel your feelings. Putting them down on paper — that's how you get to know yourself.

PRACTICE DELIGHTED LISTENING

Delighted listening uses body language that shows you are paying attention. When you use eye contact and don't interrupt, and you lean your body slightly forward, and nod or tilt your head in appropriate response, you assure the person who is talking that you are engaged in the act of listening, and you are hearing what they say. Listening is a good habit to adopt. When you listen to others, they get to know themselves and you get the credit, even though all you did was listen.

I have had people thank me for how helpful I was when I never said a word. For example, our children would come to me and say, "Dad, I've got a problem." The first time, I'd respond by giving advice such as "Okay, read this book; go see this person; take this medicine" — and they'd always say, "You're no help."

The next time they'd come to me and say, "Dad, I've got a problem," I'd ask, "What is it?" Then I'd just sit and listen for twenty minutes or half an hour, and when they were done, they'd say, "Thanks, Dad. You've been such a big help." And what did I say during all that time? Nothing more than "Hmmm" in an empathetic or understanding tone. Why did it work? Somebody had heard them.

I had one woman come to me with a problem, and I didn't say a word for ninety minutes. When she was done, she said, "That is one of the most meaningful conversations I have ever had in my life." She was talking to herself, and it was meaningful.

So, keep a journal. Listen. Pay attention to your feelings. Be authentic.

Chapter 10

WORDS CAN KILL OR CURE

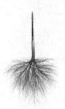

One learns that worlds are made by words
and not only hammers and wires.

— JAMES HILLMAN

*M*any years ago I was asked to see a young woman who everyone thought had appendicitis. I didn't agree with the diagnosis, and after observing her it became apparent that her problem was a ruptured ovarian cyst, which did not require surgery. A few years later, the woman's younger sister, a talented musician, tripped at home and fell into the fireplace, seriously burning her hands, arms, upper torso, and neck. When she was sent to the Yale–New Haven Hospital emergency room, the family asked me to care for her.

Her hands were disfigured, and she was seriously depressed knowing this would end her musical career. I admitted her to the hospital burn unit, and each morning I would debride her burns while she screamed at me, "I hate you." Her words really made me think about why I had become a doctor and whether I wanted to continue, if this was the reaction patients had to me when I was trying to help them heal. (Years later her mother told me that one morning I said to her, "Madeline, maybe someday you'll love me." I don't recall that moment, but knowing how I behave, I probably said that to ease my own pain and frustration.)

One summer day, when the temperature was well over ninety degrees, into my office walked Madeline for her routine visit. She was wearing a turtleneck jersey with long sleeves. I asked her why she was dressed that way on such a hot day, and she said, "Because I am ugly."

She also told me she was looking for a summer job, and I said, "Oh, I know a nursing home that needs some aides. If I can get you a job there, are you interested?" She said yes, so I worked it out and called her back a few days later to give her the information. What I knew was that she would have to wear a uniform, which would reveal all her scars to the senior citizens she cared for.

At the end of the summer, Madeline came for her office visit, and I asked her how the job had gone. She responded, "I love my job. And no one noticed my scars."

"When you are giving love, you are beautiful," I told her. She looked at me, and her eyes filled with the light of understanding.

Madeline went on to become a nurse, and shortly after she graduated I received a phone call from her. "Doctor Siegel, I am getting married, but my father died two years ago. Would you be my father at my wedding?" I can still feel the tears I shed when she asked me. After shouting words of hate at me while she was in pain, she now spoke words of love. Of course I said yes, and the greatest gift to me was when we danced after the wedding to a Kenny Rogers song, "Through the Years." It was Madeline's way of saying that over the years, especially when she struggled, I had never let her down and I had helped her turn her life around. It helped me to heal a physician's lifetime of wounds.

One guy suggested to his friend that she could change the negative things in her life by simply changing her words. He told her, "Instead of saying I *have* to pay the bills, or I *have* to go to work, try saying, I *get* to pay the bills, or I *get* to go to work." When his friend practiced doing that, she found her outlook on everything changed from one of resentment and worry into one of gratitude and grace. She realized that all aspects of her life, from tedious small tasks to big challenging difficulties, were gifts. Changing one word changed her life. One word — how powerful is that?

Many years ago one of our children brought home a canvas he had decorated in his school art class. He had filled the entire canvas with one word: words. As a surgeon, I know you can kill or cure with a sword or scalpel. But what immediately struck me about the image on canvas was that you can also kill or cure with words, when *wordswordswords* becomes *swordswordswords*.

Physicians are not taught how to communicate with patients. Because of their fear of being sued, they tell people about all the adverse side effects of therapy and never mention the benefits. Every time I hear a TV commercial mentioning how the pill being advertised can kill you, I wonder why anyone would try it. Similarly, one hospital, in order not to be sued, would tell surgical patients the risks and possible complications of surgery — just before they went into the operating room. These patients had a higher cardiac arrest rate.

I began to realize that a patient's beliefs were more important than the diagnosis. In a sense this idea is summed up by something I was told about psychiatrist Dr. Milton Erickson. He was seeing a patient who needed some positive feedback. After writing something in her chart, he excused himself and stepped out of the office for a minute, leaving her chart open on his desk. This patient peeked at the chart and read the words "Doing well." How therapeutic. Those two words would have helped her to believe in herself and given her the boost she needed to keep working.

As I learned the power of words, I began to pay more attention to what was said in the operating room, and I changed even simple things like preparing a child for an injection. Rather than say it was going to feel like a bee sting, I'd say it would be like a mosquito bite. When an anesthesiologist talked to the patient about the patient's "going out," I would ask the patient, "When was the last time you went out on a date?" and he or she would go with a smile.

During surgery I would ask my patients to divert the blood away from the area of surgery and not bleed while I was working there. Before they awakened from surgery I would say, "You will wake up comfortable, thirsty, and hungry." Later I had to amend that with: "but you won't finish what's on your plate," when my patients all began to gain weight.

What really opened my mind to the power of words was my experience as a pediatric surgeon. To reassure children that they would not be in pain when they were undergoing surgery, I would tell them while in the emergency room: "You will go to sleep when you go into the operating room." I was shocked to have children fall asleep while they were being wheeled into the OR. One boy flipped over and went to sleep as we entered the OR. When I turned him over for his appendectomy, he awakened and said, "You told me I would go to sleep, and I sleep on my stomach," so we had to reach a compromise.

Then I began therapeutically deceiving more kids by rubbing them with an alcohol sponge, prior to drawing blood, and saying, "This will numb your skin." A third of them had total anesthesia, while the others had at least a less emotional and less painful experience — and told me it didn't work. I apologized and blamed the defective alcohol sponge.

With the parent's cooperation, we also reduced the side effects of their treatment when we relabeled vitamins as hair-growing, anti-nausea, or pain pills, and the kids responded according to the label.

One woman I know was feeling nauseated after her chemo. She asked her daughter to get her a Compazine pill, since she wasn't wearing her glasses. Her daughter gave her the pill and her nausea went away. Hours later, while wearing her glasses, she asked for another pill.

When she saw it, she told her daughter, "That's not my Compazine; that's my anticoagulant, Coumadin."

"Well, Mom, it worked fine the last time I gave it to you," her daughter responded. They were impressed by the power of suggestion to make changes in the body, even when it wasn't intentional.

I'd rather tell a therapeutic lie to a patient than list the side effects of a treatment and, in doing so, induce all of them, because what people hear from an authority figure has an even greater effect. When I did have to share information about negative side effects, I would add that they didn't happen to everyone, just as not everyone is allergic to peanuts.

Our bodies respond to our beliefs. One woman was told she was terminal owing to leukemia, and that it was a waste of time to drive for hours to receive chemotherapy, since it would only make her feel worse. Her cousin, a nurse's aide, knew me and told the woman to come up to New Haven for treatment because "Doctor Siegel makes people well all the time."

I admitted the woman to the hospital not knowing about the aide's comment. I sat on the patient's bed and explained that I would ask an oncologist friend to come and see her, as I could not treat leukemia with surgery. Then I gave her a big hug and went to call the oncologist. He told me later that he agreed with her doctor about the likely outcome, but would give her treatment to make her feel there was hope. His notes to me after the chemotherapy sessions began with the comment "doing well" and ended with: "in complete remission." I heard later that she said, "When Doctor Siegel hugged me, I knew I would get well."

As I learned about the power of words, they became my therapeutic tools. Using my Paradox technique and humor, I was able to readjust people's thoughts and feelings. I was the police surgeon in New Haven, Connecticut, for many years, and I got to know many police officers through that work. One day a policeman I knew called my office. When I picked up the phone he said, "Doctor Siegel, I am going to commit suicide."

I answered, "Jimmy, if you commit suicide I will never speak to you again." He hung up the phone and fifteen minutes later was in my office, mad as hell, shouting that he had been holding a gun in his mouth and look how insensitive and uncaring I was.

"And did you notice you're not dead?" I asked. Then he laughed and we became buddies.

Do you remember when you were a child and someone called you names? You probably answered, "Sticks and stones will break my bones, but words will never hurt me." I can tell you now: that statement is not true. Words *can* hurt and do a lot of damage. Words can kill or cure. Words, particularly those spoken by the authority figures in our lives, have power to affect us and alter our lives.

How you perceive something determines how it works for you, and the choice of words used for something plays a part in your perception. Consider four chemotherapy drugs used in a protocol named after the first letter of each drug: EPOH. One oncologist noted that if you turned the letters around, it became HOPE. He changed the name for his patients, and more of them responded to therapy.

A child's drawing was criticized by her first grade teacher, who said it would not be displayed with the others because of how she used the color purple. In second grade, when asked by another teacher to draw a picture, the child left her paper blank. This teacher came over, placed his hand on her head, and said, "The snowfall — how clean, white, and beautiful!" His words gave her permission to be creative again, and that event later inspired her to write a poem titled "Purple." You can read Alexis Rotella's poem in my book *Love, Magic & Mudpies*.

Animals, too, are subject to our perceptions based on words. One family adopted an older rescued cat who had been so traumatized by his experiences with people that he would never enter a room with people in it. He came out to eat only when the family went to bed. After several unsuccessful months of trying to gain his confidence, they consulted an animal intuitive and told her the cat's name was Spooky.

"Change his name to something macho," she suggested. "You may be projecting your expectation of his fear by the name you gave him."

They renamed the cat Rambo. Almost immediately the cat's behavior began to change. The family reported that Rambo was not only hanging around the house when they were awake, but he also had taken to sleeping on their beds at night instead of staying downstairs.

When Betty Croker was diagnosed with Stage IV breast cancer in 1962, her doctor told her the cancer was terminal. "How long do I have?" she asked. "Six months" was his reply. Imagine the impact his words had on her. Her two little girls would soon become motherless. Betty went home prepared to die, but her husband said they should ask for a second opinion.

Betty's husband went to the Yale Cancer Center and asked for a doctor on the oncology team to see his wife. While she was undergoing more tests, Betty recounted how she and her husband had fallen in love at a big band swing dance. She reminisced about the fun she and Fred used to have at their favorite dance club, and how everyone else would clear the floor so they could watch the couple dance.

Betty kept up a cheerful front throughout the testing procedures and after, as they waited for results, but Fred knew she was terrified for her two girls. She admitted to him that the first doctor's words "terminal" and "six months" had nearly taken all her hope of survival. I have seen people die in a week when hope was taken away.

When they sat down with the Yale oncologist, the doctor looked at her and smiled. "Betty, you will not be dying in six months," he said. "In six months, we will have you dancing again."

The doctor's words gave her hope. Six months to the day, Betty put on a new dress and wore her red dancing shoes. Her girls watched with excitement as their parents got ready for their big night out. Years later, I had the opportunity to work with one of Betty's daughters. She told me, "I still remember how happy Dad was and how beautiful Mom looked that night. They were like a couple of kids going out on their first date. That doctor gave my mom permission to live," she said. "I'm sure it was because of him that we had her for three more years. I will never be able to thank him enough."

From "terminal" and "six months" to "dancing" and "you'll live" — that's the power of words. If your doctor or health practitioner doesn't believe in your recovery, fire him or her. Find someone who believes in miracles — someone who believes in you.

AFFIRMATIONS

A coach encourages his team with phrases such as *You can do it* and *Go out there and live up to your potential* because he knows his words will ring in the minds of his players when they face their opponents. His encouragement can make or break the team's spirit, and that is often the decisive factor in whether or not they give it their best effort.

A good coach realizes that the key is to know that you did your best, and that you are not a loser if you don't win the game. Losers are afraid to take a chance, whether facing a disease or another opponent, and they live with guilt, blame, and shame. Don't empower your enemies by focusing on fighting and beating them, but *empower your effort* by giving it your best shot and believing in yourself.

The most effective affirmations are short, positive statements that, like mantras, are easily remembered, and that state something as if it has already happened. Instead of "I will recover from this cancer," a more effective affirmation would be: "My body is glowing with health." This statement allows you to see your true potential, your divine nature, and focuses not on what is wrong but on what is right within you. When you imagine it, your body responds as if it is already happening.

Our creator has built into all living things the ability to survive. Wounds heal, bacteria resist antibiotics, viruses resist antivirals, and trees resist parasites, all because we have the ability to alter our genes and survive. Your body needs to know that you love it, and love your life, to make the necessary survival effort.

Identify the negative statements you may hold in your mind. Write a positive affirmation for each one that helps you to turn the negative thought around. If you are worrying about something or unsuccess-fully trying to control people and situations, try using the affirmation "Let go and let God." If you are struggling with any major challenge, try: "One day at a time." Merely the act of writing the affirmation "Just for today I will…" (for example, "stay sober" or "practice listening") produces strong momentum in the intention behind your decision to behave differently. If you struggle with self-esteem, try using: "I am perfect just the way I am." If you struggle with self-confidence, write: "I achieve whatever I set my heart on."

Remember, this will not set you up for failure if you don't live up to your affirmation. Your goal is to fake it till you make it. Act and behave as if you are the person you want to become, and keep rehearsing. Find life coaches, too, to help you practice.

Sometimes a single word painted on the wall or etched in a stone is a powerful affirmation. Words such as *Faith, Peace, Gratitude, Laughter,* and *Beloved* can help you to love yourself better. Fill your home and workplace with these. Our house is filled with mottoes to live by. One example of a good life motto is a quote of Lao Tzu: "Be content with what you have; rejoice in the way things are. When you realize there is nothing lacking, the whole world belongs to you."[1] You can also put up the serenity prayer and practice reading it out loud. Keep a deck of affirmation cards handy, and treat yourself several times a day. Even the words of a song can soothe, encourage, and inspire.

So get creative, buy some paint, and stencil a loving message to yourself on the wall you walk by most often. I have a portrait of my parents on my wall so that they are always watching me, and I don't want to disappoint them. Put a welcome sign above the bathroom mirror, look into your eyes every morning, and greet yourself with: "Hi, sunshine. Welcome to today!"

With every dawn that you wake up to, you are like a blank canvas. Just as nature paints the horizon, you are creating a work of art, so always have more colors on the palette, and keep retouching your work until you are satisfied with the results.

SUBLIMINAL AFFIRMATIONS

A still, calm mind has a better chance of clearly reflecting on an issue and coming up with a remedy. If you need help getting started, you can use a CD I created just for this purpose: *Finding Your True Self: Audible and Subliminal Affirmations to Develop Your Personal Sense of Inner Peace and Wisdom.* Research studies show that subliminal affirmations and meditations are an easy and effective way to overcome mental hurdles and to give yourself better health and happiness throughout your life. Choose a specific time and a quiet, undisturbed place for your therapy. When you encounter stressful situations, you can call upon this inner peace immediately, stopping stress in its tracks.

DANCE A NEW DANCE

Negative words and images fill our minds at such an early age that it takes conscious effort to later change those habits of belief. Sometimes we carry a feeling of self-pity as well, believing we are not good enough or we don't deserve to be happy. When this happens, we need to play a different tape, learn a new song, and dance a new dance.

Sharon had been raised in a home where her mother's mental illness prevented her from giving Sharon messages of love, messages that would build self-worth and self-esteem. While Sharon was eventually able to understand and forgive her mother, she found it impossible to believe in her own worthiness, to see herself as someone who deserved love. When we internalize our negative feelings and try to please everyone else in order to feel valuable, we lose our authentic lives. So it did not surprise me that Sharon developed breast cancer at a young age and underwent a mastectomy followed by chemotherapy, or that the depression she experienced during and after this was almost overwhelming.

As a doctor, I can tell you that her low feelings of self-worth threatened her life more than any cancer or chemotherapy drug. One day

Sharon's therapist suggested that she list her daily blessings. Every time someone showed a kindness, she should write it down. If someone called or sent a card, or even if a stranger opened a door for her or put a quarter in her parking meter — no matter how big or how small the kindness — she was supposed to write it down.

Sharon bought a journal and began keeping track of the thoughtful, kind things people said and did for her. The more she noticed the kindnesses, the more positive she felt. She began doing kind things for others as well, sometimes when they knew about it, and often when they didn't. As the weeks and months went by, Sharon filled page after page, not only with kindnesses, but also with all the blessings in her life. Two years after her mastectomy, with a clean bill of health, Sharon read through her journals, realizing how lucky she was not only to have regained her health but also for how loved she felt. She had gained a large measure of self-worth. She knows that when she walks into a room these days, people are genuinely happy to see her. Listing the positives instead of focusing on the negatives completely turned her life around.

Studies have shown that when one person engages in a kind act for another person or an animal, both the doer and the receiver experience a warm sense of belonging caused by the release of endorphins and bonding hormones, feel-good chemicals that make your body want to live. Not only do the giver and receiver benefit, but so do the observers of a kindness, who receive the same chemical burst. It is like taking a lit candle into a darkened room. The candle glows within its own aura, but the whole room receives a portion of its light.

ADOPT A DIFFERENT ATTITUDE

If each of us is here on earth to give our soul an opportunity to grow and to be of service to those whose lives are touched by ours, then it makes sense to adopt an attitude that helps us to achieve this end. When you are having difficulties, and you ask yourself, "What am I to learn from this experience?" things will change for you. These feelings and events will lead you to find nourishment for yourself and your life. And when you love your life and body, your body will do all it can to keep you alive. Another way to approach things when you are suffering any kind of physical discomfort, pain, or emotional turmoil is to ask yourself: "What has to change in order for me to change this experience?"

Sometimes the change we need to make involves being emotionally honest with ourselves. A good example of emotional dishonesty is when you are asked to go to a social event, or to take on a new responsibility, and your mind is thinking, "No, I don't want to do that," but your mouth says, "Yes, okay." There is a difference between submissiveness and politeness. Trying to be a people-pleaser can get you into trouble. Remember that, just as expressing appropriate anger is beneficial, you also have the right to say no to the things you do not want to do. I like to remember that an English teacher once told me, " 'No' is a complete sentence." It is a wonderful feeling of empowerment when you learn to say no. Rather than going to the event you do not wish to attend, learn to say, "Thank you. I won't be coming, but I appreciate your thoughtfulness for inviting me." To the person who pressures you to take on another commitment, learn to say, "Thank you for asking, but no. I am fully committed." If they catch you at a weak moment and you have difficulty saying no, use another tack. Tell the person you need to think about it and will let them know. Then find someone you can rehearse your responses with. As soon as you can, call the other person back or send an email. Don't let others decide your life. You decide what you want. Let your heart make up your mind.

DOCTOR'S R_x

Notice how often you say "I have to" or "I should." Every time you hear yourself using these words, repeat the statement, but change "I have to" or "I should" to "I get to." Notice how different each expression makes you feel. Describe those feelings in your journal. For example:

"I have to pay the bills" makes me feel anxious, pressured.

"I get to pay the bills" makes me feel grateful, empowered.

Make a habit of doing this every day for one month, and watch what happens to your outlook and overall mood. Stay aware of the language you use, and incorporate positive words into your daily thinking and speaking, so the "I can't"s become "I can"s.

Chapter 11

CHOOSE LIFE

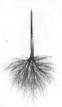

When your answer is "world peace," you will find inner peace.
Transcend the personal and choose life for everyone.

— BERNIE SIEGEL

I believe that much of my reverence for life and living beings came from my father's appreciation for the truly important things: trust, faith, hope, and love. My father was only twelve when he learned just how precious and precarious life is. He lost his father to an untimely death from tuberculosis, one that left my grandmother and her six children in a desperate situation.

Life is not unfair but it is difficult. Becoming strong at the broken places is neither easy nor fun. We are constantly being tested by both positive and negative situations and circumstances. And it is this testing process that tempers and strengthens us if we adopt life-enhancing attitudes and behavior. This decision to choose what is best for our lives often doesn't happen until we find ourselves stricken with cancer or other disease, facing divorce, or experiencing loss of some kind.

When we become stuck in a pattern of living only for our children or our spouse, or even for the company that employs us, we deviate from our true path. We all need to live our authentic, unique lives and not fulfill a role. I knew a mother of nine who said, "I can't die till they're all married and out of the house." When her ninth kid left home twenty years later, her cancer returned and she died. Rather than live for your kids, live for the child inside you. Then when your kids leave home, you won't die from a life that no longer has meaning for you.

One of the miracles of life is that we can choose at any time to get back on the path to fulfill our purpose for living. You might well ask, "How do I do that?"

This doesn't mean we should give up our families and stop working, but that we should find a balance between doing for others and doing for ourselves. When you find meaning in your life and learn to say yes to what makes you happy, and no to the things you do not want to do, life becomes easier to survive. Then we are prepared to take less money for the right job or take a risk and do something we are passionate about.

You have to start with a belief in yourself, have faith in all the things you incorporate into your life, and, when you are ill, believe in the things you choose as therapy. You need to be in touch with your inner desires and greater self. I see it as having the right Lord and giving love in your chosen way. Your focus then is on living a healed life rather than avoiding death.

Karen and her husband had high-paying careers in the finance industry until her husband, who was only in his forties, became ill with so-called terminal cancer. They took early retirement, sold their apartment, bought some land and started a berry farm. It was something they had talked about doing when they retired, but after the cancer treatment, they decided it was now or never. Fifteen years later, Karen and her husband are running a successful berry farm and sell their berry preserves and marinades all over the world. By taking a risk in a leap of faith, they proved to themselves that when you live in your heart, miracles happen.

I am often reminded of the biblical message that says when life (and good) and death (and evil) are placed before us, we are to choose life. This does not mean simply that we should try to avoid dying. We should choose to live a meaningful life that involves us in a demonstration of love for ourselves and others. When we live that way, our bodies know we love life, and they do all they can to sustain us, heal our afflictions and wounds, and keep us healthy mentally and physically. Remember, as I've said before, your thoughts and feelings create your internal chemistry. A patient of mine, a landscaper who was about to retire, refused treatment for his cancer after surgery because it was springtime and he wanted to go home and make the world beautiful before he died. He lived to be ninety-four and became my teacher about what it means to choose life and not be focused on what is good for only you.

We now know from scientific studies how one's emotions and personality affect survival rates. We understand that simple things like laughter affect the survival of cancer patients, and that meaningless retirement and loneliness affect the genes that control immune function. I also believe there are other factors that *help* us, and these are greater than we can possibly imagine. Some call these miracles, luck, serendipity, or just being in the right place at the right time. When everything falls into place and seeming coincidences appear with perfect timing, this synchronicity of events suggests there is a loving intelligence that is beyond our capacity to understand, but not beyond our ability to experience. I know people who have left their troubles to God and have been cured of cancer.

You don't have to wait until you are sick and your existence is threatened before you start to live your authentic life with trust and faith. Listening to your intuition and acting on it will bring you unexpected gifts at any time in your life.

It was in 1997 when William and Danielle from Laguna Hills, California, learned they were expecting their first child. Danielle believed that the attitudes she adopted throughout pregnancy would affect the child inside her, and so she determined to remain positive and to pay attention to her instincts. When choosing an obstetrician-gynecologist from the Laguna Hills obstetric practices, Danielle scrolled down the list of available doctors, and her finger stopped at a Dr. Blake Spring (name changed to protect confidentiality). "I know this sounds a bit crazy," she confessed to William. "But I have such a strong feeling about this doctor — something tells me he's the right one for us."

"When your wife makes a decision like that, especially when she's pregnant," William told me, "it's best to go along for the ride."

Danielle called the doctor's office and made an appointment. Before her first visit with Dr. Spring, she searched through the drawer for her medical records and happened upon William's birth certificate. She was surprised to see the attending physician who signed William's birth certificate in 1974 was also a Dr. Blake Spring, but at a different hospital.

When Danielle and William went for their first consultation at Saddleback Memorial Medical Center, they handed William's birth certificate to Dr. Spring and asked if that was his signature. "It certainly is," he said with a grin. "Riverside Hospital was where I did my ob/gyn internship. You were one of the first babies I delivered." Danielle felt it was a good omen that the doctor who helped her husband into this world would now do the same for their first baby.

Months later Danielle delivered a healthy baby, having experienced no complications during pregnancy or the birth. William's mother came and was delighted to reconnect with the doctor who had delivered her son. Everyone agreed afterwards that, throughout Danielle's labor and delivery, it felt like a happy family reunion. Right from the start, the couple felt as if a greater hand had been directing them every step of the way. By listening to her intuition, Danielle and William had allowed synchronicity to play its harmonious role in the joy-filled birth of their first child.

Danielle was motivated to remain positive because she was doing it for her baby. But we can do this for ourselves too. Once when I was feeling troubled by difficult circumstances that I found myself in, I telephoned a friend, and she asked, "Bernie, do you get upset when you're hungry?"

"No, I get something to eat."

Then she told me to ask myself: What nourishment do I need? What can I do with my life to take away the feelings I don't like about this situation or this moment? These questions are powerful because they make you stop and think about your life: What do I need to change or bring into my life? How does this curse I'm living with become a blessing? When you use whatever affliction you have and learn from it, the challenge becomes your teacher. And it changes your attitude toward it, so even if something can't be cured, you can still heal and be a teacher for others with the same problem. Some people describe their curse as the catalyst for a new beginning, their wake-up call, or a blessing in disguise.

Animals that lose a body part don't go and hide in the corner because they don't look normal. But people who are disfigured or seriously injured often experience anger and shame, thinking they are no longer beautiful or functional. This thinking is faulty, but people can change their thinking.

Several years ago I met a woman who had been born without arms as a result of her mother taking the prescription drug thalidomide for nausea during pregnancy. When I saw this woman in a cafeteria using her feet to put dishes on her tray, and people carrying it to the table for her, I went to sit with her. I said, "I'd like to learn from you, about your attitude, the way you deal with life's difficulties, and more."

She said, "Give me the pen," and wrote down all her contact information with a pen between her toes.

Even though I couldn't cure her and she couldn't cure herself, she was already healed. She was a gift to others and a teacher to me. She, like Helen Keller, became my coach. She wasn't sitting home feeling bitter or resentful at her parents and God, saying, "Look what they did to me." No, she chose life and learned what she could do with the body she had.

When you make the choice to focus on solutions rather than the problem — under any circumstances — it becomes life enhancing for you as well as for others. It's not a selfish choice, and it helps you to find nourishment.

It's easy to tell people to choose life. But how do you know when something is the right choice or is God's will for you? When a Catholic nun was asked the question "How do you know what God's will is?" she replied, "I know what God's will is not. When I find myself pushing a pea uphill with my nose, and the pea keeps rolling down the hill, that is not God's will."

My mother's answer to that question was more direct. She always used to say, "Do what will make you happy." By saying this, she taught me to stay in touch with my feelings.

I asked a group of people once: "If you had only fifteen minutes to live, what would you do?" There were all kinds of answers, from playing golf and working in the garden, to calling loved ones and so on. When our son said, "I'd buy a quart of chocolate ice cream and eat it," I told him, "I don't have to worry about you — you're enlightened."

Then somebody said, "Wait a minute — you didn't like my answer, but what if the thing I chose to do is my equivalent to chocolate ice cream?"

Fair enough, I thought. So now I say to people, "Find your chocolate ice cream." Find what makes you lose track of time. That's the healthiest state you can ever be in. I know this from personal experience. You are totally unaware of your body; you're free of pain, free of disease, because you're doing something creative. I found I could stand in the operating room for hours, even with a back injury, and have no problem; I could paint a portrait standing in front of an easel and not be aware of my back. But when those activities ended, I was either on the floor or on the sofa because anywhere else was too painful.

When you're doing something you love to do, your body chemistry changes — your body gets the message. I have another story that illustrates how well this works. Not only is Bath, England, a popular destination for tourists, but it is also a major center for arthritis research, at the Royal National Hospital for Rheumatic Diseases. Years ago a friend of mine owned a gift shop near the hospital. One day, after returning from a buying trip, she created a window display with a large selection of handblown glass. As she said in a note to me later,

> I displayed all the green, turquoise, and cyan blue bowls, jugs, plates, and vases, until they filled the whole window. When I turned the spotlights on and the light shone through the colored glass, it looked like a tropical ocean wave, with the deeper colors on the bottom and the lighter ones at the top. After I finished the display, a lady with a cane stopped to gaze at the window. I was pleased that she seemed to enjoy my creative work, but half an hour later she was still standing there gazing, and I began to wonder if there was something wrong with her. I went out and asked if she was okay. She then told me that for many years she had been suffering chronic pain from rheumatoid arthritis, but while she looked at the beautiful greens and blues, time disappeared, and the pain had totally left her. She said she hadn't felt that well in years. I will never forget the look of peace on her face.

By being grateful and nourishing her soul with something beautiful, this woman gave her body what it needed. Time no longer had any meaning. She chose to live her life, instead of living and being her illness, and in doing so she found relief from pain.

Decades ago, before tape recorders were allowed in the operating room, I brought them in to play music because it helped my patients to relax. I chose something that made me feel better too. At first the staff said, "That's not hospital policy — it's a hazard around the explosive anesthetic gases," but when everyone felt better from listening to the peaceful music, they stopped complaining. Today we have studies verifying the benefits of music — it shortens the length of time needed for the surgery, patients require less anesthesia, and they have less postoperative pain.

My prescription for choosing life and finding your true path is to use love as your motivation and inspiration. So do what you love to do, and find your own way of contributing your love to the world. Be with those who accept you as you are. Be accepting of those you meet. Love is blind, because it does not see faults in others. It also helps us to heal past differences and maintain healthy relationships. I like the following prayer: "Dear God, teach me to treat people today the way I hope you will treat me tomorrow." The attitude sought in this prayer teaches us life-enhancing behavior.

I once heard a Franciscan monk tell an old story about Saint Francis and his student, Brother Leo. It was a hard winter in the hills of Italy, and they had been making a long journey on foot. As they walked in silence, they contemplated their reading from the morning, a meditation about the secret of achieving perfect joy. Brother Leo turned to Francis and asked him, "What is the secret of perfect joy?"

After explaining that people think pleasant or enlightening events will help them find joy, only to discover they don't, Saint Francis pointed across the wide, snowy valley and said, "Suppose we go to that monastery across the field and tell the gatekeeper how weary and cold we are. Then suppose he calls us tramps and beats us and throws us out into the winter night. Then, if we can say to him with love in our hearts, 'Bless you in the name of Jesus,' only then shall we have found the secret of perfect joy."

Letting go of expectations and resentments, and accepting whatever comes your way as merely the next step on your path, you will turn away from suffering and disease and will walk in health and peace.

When you can love the unlovable and forgive the unforgivable, you will be free.

Sometimes the choices other people make can have a remarkable effect on us, especially when those choices are made with love. A woman patient used to vomit after her chemotherapy; and so when she and her husband got to the car, he would hand her a bag that she could throw up in as he drove her home. One day at our support group, she was all smiles. When I asked her why, she said, "My husband handed me the bag, and when I opened it I discovered he had placed a dozen roses inside." She never needed to vomit again after her therapy.

Choosing life is a conscious choice. It is not about the luck of the draw, but a conscious decision to think and behave in such a way that your mind and body are not in conflict. One of my patients had no side effects from radiation, and the radiation therapist thought his machine was malfunctioning — until he saw my name in her chart. He told me that was when he realized: "This is one of Siegel's crazy patients." When he asked her why she had no side effects, she said to him, "I get out of the way and let the radiation go to my tumor."

I've mentioned patients who left their troubles to God and had their cancers disappear. This was due to the state of peace, tranquility, and love they had attained. It's called self-induced healing and is not a spontaneous remission. Personality characteristics and our potential to survive are inseparable. In one study that used personality profiles, psychologist Bruno Klopfer correctly predicted nineteen out of twenty-four times which patients would have fast-growing cancers and which would have cancers that grew slowly.[1]

I encourage health practitioners to learn about survival behavior from exceptional patients, by asking them why they didn't die, rather than say what doctors tend to say, which is: "You are doing very well. Whatever you're doing, keep it up." Those doctors learn nothing from these patients that they can pass on to other patients. It is vitally important for health practitioners to teach, and remind, patients of their potential.

I also remind people that relationships keep us alive, and that we need to foster a good relationship with our self as well, so that when we are alone we are not lonely. As a patient we have a responsibility to take charge of our body and our care. That means we need to teach our doctor and health care practitioners what patients are experiencing. When your doctor does not understand your point of view, tell her and teach her. If she listens and apologizes, stick with her and help her to learn from your experience. If she makes excuses or blames you, find another doctor. This is another example of how to choose life. Being a submissive sufferer and "good" patient is not survival behavior. You want to be known as a person and not as a disease or hospital room number.

Our Creator built survival mechanisms into all living things so we can heal wounds, alter our genes, and overcome various diseases. Living beings were designed to live. So be alive. Love your life and your body, and amazing things can happen.

DOCTOR'S R_x

Take the Immune-Competent Personality Test, based on Dr. George Solomon's research:

1. Do I have a sense of meaning in my work, daily activities, family, and relationships?
2. Am I able to express anger appropriately in defense of myself?
3. Am I able to ask friends and family for support when I am feeling lonely or troubled?
4. Am I able to ask friends or family for favors when I need them?
5. Am I able to say no to someone who asks for a favor if I can't do it or don't feel like doing it?

6. Do I engage in health-related behaviors based on my own self-defined needs instead of someone else's prescriptions or ideas?

7. Do I have enough play in my life?

8. Do I find myself depressed for long periods, during which time I feel hopeless about ever changing the conditions that cause me to be depressed?

9. Am I dutifully filling a prescribed role in my life to the detriment of my own needs?

ANSWERS:

If you answered yes to questions 1 through 7 and no to questions 8 and 9, you have an immune-competent personality that helps you to stay healthy, to overcome disease, and face challenges when they happen. If you answered no to the first seven questions and yes to the last two, you need to pay attention to your behavior and rebirth yourself. Most people who take this test will find they have at least some room for growth. When this happens, try adopting new attitudes and behaviors that help you to create a new person, and don't limit yourself. I even recommend choosing a new name for this new you.

Siegel's three additions to the Immune-Competent Personality Test:

1. I am taking you to dinner. Where do you want to go?

2. What would you hold up before an audience to demonstrate the beauty and meaning of life?

3. How would you introduce yourself to God?

ANSWERS:

1. Your response should relate to *your* feelings, not what it costs or the food preferences of the other person. Be

willing to accept the gift without responding to their question, "What do *you* want?"

2. A mirror.
3. By responding, "It's you" or, "Your child is here." The best answer God ever heard from a high school student was "Tell God his replacement is here."

You can find the online version of this test on my website at http://berniesiegelmd.com/resources/organizations-websites/immune-competent-personality-test/.

Chapter 12

END-OF-LIFE TRANSITIONS

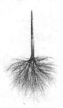

If you would indeed behold the spirit of death,
open your heart wide unto the body of life.
For life and death are one, even as the river and the sea are one.

— KAHLIL GIBRAN

I have come to understand that I am like water. Just as streams of water find their way over and around obstacles to rejoin the sea of life, I find my path in life and flow with it; and when I become vapor or mist, I will return to earth as rain does and be born again. Then, if I learn what I am here to learn, I will help to teach others how to become cocreators of a world filled with faith, hope, and love for all things.

Every life is like a candle, and the length of the candle doesn't depend on our age but on what we are scheduled to do on this planet. Our job while we are here is to illuminate the path for our self and others — not to worry about how much time we have left, but to get the job done. We need to burn up, rather than burn out before our time.

As George Bernard Shaw said, "Life is no brief candle to me, it is a sort of splendid torch which I've got hold of for a moment, and I want to make it burn as brightly as possible before handing it on to future generations."[1]

When a person develops a life-threatening illness such as cancer, family members also become afflicted by the experience, which they are rarely prepared for. Not only must they deal with grief from the expectation of loss, but also they will be faced with caring for the dying person while the latter undergoes treatment, a person whose needs can impose demands on many levels. Unless the family has already lived through and learned from a previous loss, this period of transition is not something you can prepare for, in the sense that your feelings and experiences will happen when they happen and not before.

Financial responsibilities, role changes, and physical, mental, and emotional energy demands all have the potential to become overwhelming at this time. People who deal with illness in the family only on an intellectual level may appear to be coping well, but ignoring their own feelings and needs can send them to the sickbed, too. Statistics show that the people who care for chronically or terminally ill patients frequently succumb to illness or death before, or shortly after, the patient dies, because they stop taking care of their own physical and emotional needs.

Self-care has to be a priority, and this can happen in many ways. Accepting help from others, taking breaks, joining support groups, enjoying laughter clubs or funny movies, eating well, maintaining some way of listening to the inner voice, talking to God, and letting God talk back — these are all lifesaving measures that help people through the stages of letting their loved ones go while caring for them as long as they are alive. The song *Rock Me to Sleep*, written by Tom Hunter, and which I mentioned in chapter 9, says it well in the chorus: "Tonight I'd like you to rock me to sleep; I'd like you to sing me a song; I'm tired of doing things all by myself, and I'm tired of being so strong."[2] Looking after yourself stems from self-love, because if you do not value yourself the experience will become self-destructive and will not be life enhancing for anyone involved.

The important thing for caregivers to remember is to seek help before a disaster awakens you. You do not have to become strong at the broken places. You can learn how to handle the difficult elements of life just as a tree survives changes in the weather. When a patient is doing creative therapies to deal with their disease, family members can do the same, getting as much benefit as the patient does by working with their own unconscious through the use of imagery, drawings, and other forms of creative expression, such as playing music or journaling. It helps family members to identify what they fear and how they feel, so they can seek help through grief counseling or support groups. The hospice movement also provides support for family members, including counseling for up to a year after the patient dies, and many organized religions and churches offer similar help.

When a terminally ill patient is working with drawings, he who no longer finds his body an enjoyable place to be, and whose will to live no longer exists, will often draw his impending death without realizing he is doing so. This may take the form of a purple butterfly or balloon rising into the sky. Another sign may be that his drawings done over a period of time are showing lighter, fading colors, alerting the family that it may be time to talk about it.

Family members may feel uncomfortable talking with the dying person about the end of life and afterward, but it can be very helpful for both if they do so. Open discussion on these matters by asking the patient questions such as "What are you thinking?" and "How are you feeling?" Bringing up the subject is okay. If the patient doesn't want to discuss it, he'll shut you off. Creative imagery can also be used to open discussion. Asking the patient to close his eyes and imagine how he would feel in a totally white room usually gets a positive response from those who need a rest or are ready for a spiritual transition. Those who are not ready to die are bored with the image of white walls and want to leave that room or decorate it.

Speaking up about your own needs and feelings regarding the upcoming transition is also appropriate when the patient is willing to listen. You can speak about your needs and see if he will speak about his, and if he does, you end up coaching and helping each other. When family members get over their fear of discussing the future with the person who is dying, and that person is ready to talk about it, wonderful things can happen. It is in these moments that our immortality is created.

A few years ago, Will was living in an AIDS hospice in Sacramento when his body systems began to shut down. My friend Jean, a volunteer grief counselor at the hospice, suggested to Will's brother that now was the time to ask Will any questions he might have, such as "How will I know you are okay after you've gone?" and "How will I know when you are with me?"

Two weeks later, as Jean prepared to go to Will's memorial service and funeral, she heard someone at her front door, but when she opened it no one was there. On the doorstep, she found three tail feathers from a blue jay. Jean picked them up and put them in her purse after admiring the perfect, striking blue feathers. As she drove to the church, she turned on the radio, and a symphony she had never heard was playing. It had a beautiful melody and playful lightness that lifted her feelings of sadness over Will's death. When the piece finished playing, the radio announcer said that the symphony, by Ottorino Respighi, was called *The Birds*.

Later, when the memorial service was over, Will's brother approached Jean. "Thank you for your advice," he said. "The day you talked with us, I asked my brother how I would know when he was with me after he died, and he told me he'd send a bird, a beautiful, bright blue bird. He even laughed and said that he would make the bird talk to me. This morning when I walked to my car, a blue jay landed at my feet, started flapping its wings, and screamed at me, so there was no way I could ignore it. I suddenly remembered Will's promise to send me a bright blue, talking bird, and the moment I realized it was Will, the bird flew off. I've felt his presence with me ever since."

Jean pulled the feathers out of her purse and gave them to Will's brother. Then she told him about the noise at her front door and the symphony on the radio. As they stood there talking, Will's mother approached holding a large bouquet of bright blue iris. The flowers were the same shade of blue as the jay's tail feathers. "I don't know who sent these," she said. "Just as we were leaving the house, a florist's van pulled up and they handed me this bouquet. They forgot to include a card."

Will's brother exchanged glances with Jean. "They're from Will," he said to his mother. "He's telling us he's okay."

If you are skeptical, let me share some of my personal experiences and what ultimately convinced a skeptical scientist like me that consciousness does not cease to exist even though a person's body has died. When I was speaking to support groups for parents whose children had died, I heard many stories that they did not feel safe sharing with most people. .

One was told to me by a woman whose son had died. His favorite bird was a seagull. She said, "I was driving on the parkway one winter when a seagull landed in the road in front of me. I could hear my son saying, 'Mom, slow down.' I stopped and the gull flew off. I started to move ahead again, slowly, and as I came around a turn in the highway, there was a sheet of ice. Many cars had already collided with one another after skidding on the ice. If I hadn't slowed down when I heard my son's voice, I would have skidded into them, too."

A father told me of his son who had died and who loved butterflies. The summer after his son's death, the father was walking in the woods near his Connecticut home when a beautiful, enormous butterfly began to follow him wherever he went. He felt it was his son coming back to help him deal with his grief. When he got home he looked through his son's books to identify the butterfly that followed him, and he found that the species existed only in South America.

Our cancer support group was meeting, and one woman mentioned that her daughter had been murdered. She shared this because she felt it was related to her becoming ill. Then she went on to say that her daughter loved birds, and that at her younger sister's outdoor wedding a bird had landed in the tree and interrupted the wedding with its loud call. Everyone at the wedding said to her, "Your daughter's here." As she finished telling us the story, a bird flew into the open window, and of course we reacted as they had at the wedding. In all the years we had been in that room, no bird had even landed on the windowsill, let alone entered the room.

Several times while I have been lecturing, insects have flown around my shaved head while I stood on the stage speaking. Usually I wave at them once to see what their intentions are. If they remain after a wave, I know they are looking for a warm, loving place to land and renew themselves. I explain this to the audience so they are not distracted by the insect sitting on my shaved head while I continue to speak. When the insect is a wasp, the audience is naturally concerned, but from my communication with the wasp, I know I have nothing to fear. I have learned to listen to what they have to say, even though they are not speaking in words. Their thoughts are received by me and mine by them when I can keep my mind quiet and free of turbulence, like a still pond.

I show slides during my lectures, and one is a picture of a butterfly sitting on my wife's shoulder. Many years ago a patient of mine went to the island of Kauai in Hawaii to die, because her mother lived there and she wanted to heal her relationship with her mother before she died. Several years later I was invited to speak and present a workshop in Kauai.

While staying on the island, Bobbie and I went shopping, and as we entered a store, Bobbie noticed a tiger swallowtail butterfly trapped in a large chandelier. It seemed confused by all the lights. Bobbie's reverence for life made her feel the need to rescue it, so she climbed up on the counter and held out her hand to the butterfly. It flew onto her palm and she climbed down. We went outside to release it, but it wouldn't leave. If we brushed it off one shoulder, it flew to the other or to her hand. So we stopped trying to brush it off and let it accompany us.

That night I said, "Bobbie, you need to let the butterfly go. We'll crush it if we take it to bed with us." She went out on the porch, returned, and said, "I brushed it off my shoulder." I said, "Honey, now it's sitting on your other shoulder." We finally arranged a plate of sweet water on a kitchen counter, and the butterfly settled on the plate rim for the evening.

The next day after breakfast, it hopped onto Bobbie again. I put it in a paper bag and took it to the outdoor workshop with us, planning to use it as part of my talk about transformation and about life being a series of beginnings and not endings. After discussing the symbolism of the butterfly freeing itself from the caterpillar's cocoon, I opened the bag and let our butterfly out to demonstrate. It spent the day overhead and did not leave until after the workshop finished. That butterfly had spent fourteen hours with my wife, not counting the workshop. Why? Who was it? My answer is that it represented the spirit and conscious-ness of my patient, and that was her way of thanking me and saying good-bye.

One woman wrote to me asking how to deal with her grief over the death of her parents. She said she just couldn't get used to the fact they were no longer there. She still had her Mom's number on her phone, and all she wanted to do was call her again and say all the things she never did.

I wrote back to her suggesting that she read my book *Buddy's Can-dle* and learn what her parents wanted for her. The story helps people realize that consciousness doesn't end, and we can still talk to our par-ents. You may hear them answer, or may have a dream in which they talk to you, or you might find meaningful things around the house and garden that make you realize they're with you. Your loved ones do not want you to grieve and diminish your joy in living. They want you to enjoy the day and not have your tears put out their celestial candle of life.

I went through the same feeling this woman did, and yes, I used to dial my mom's number, wanting to tell her something and forgetting that she had died. But now I have a portrait of my parents in the front hall and their photo on my computer as the screen saver, so they are always with me. You can create similar shrines around your house, too.

Children and teens who suffer the loss of a parent need help dealing with their grief. One teenage boy seemed to be coping well with the loss of his dad. His mother depended on him for helping with the other children, and he had never let her down. A year after his father died, however, he suddenly started acting out and skipping school. His grades suffered, and he quit participating in his favorite sports. Suspecting this was a delayed reaction to losing his dad, the boy's mother enrolled him in a grief therapy group for teens. They listened to music, made drawings, and talked about their feelings. The boy never said much in the group until one day when the other kids called him on it. They asked him what he was holding back, because he always seemed so angry with them and wouldn't open up.

The boy finally told them that about a year after his dad died, he had picked up the mail, and a pamphlet from their church was included in it. On the back were listed the church board members, one of whom had been his father, but somebody had crossed his dad's name off with a black felt-tip pen. "When I saw that black mark over Dad's name, it really hit me — he's dead," said the teen as tears started rolling down his cheeks. "I was so angry. After everything Dad did for the church, somebody had picked up a pen and blacked out his name like it didn't matter, like he'd never existed." The other kids listened quietly and did not try to stop him from crying, for they had learned that healing tears were what he needed. Afterward, when they talked with him he seemed much more relaxed and ready to join the group. That was the beginning of his journey through the grief, and his mom reported that his attitude improved and his grades at school went back up again.

When you lose somebody, celebrate your love for them and theirs for you. Keep the dialogue open about the person who died, especially with your kids, so they don't think their loved one has been forgotten or crossed off. Remind the kids that the person is perfect again, and they can still share their thoughts and feelings with them; the loved one's spirit will know. The only thing in this life that is immortal is love, and love is your bridge to this individual forever.

I have no problem sharing with you that I have heard the voices of dead patients and family members speaking to me. I have also had mystics bring me messages from my dead patients and family members, and in doing so these mystics have used those individuals' names and characteristic expressions when talking.

One last personal story: Elisabeth Kübler-Ross, as I mentioned, was a very good friend and a teacher of mine. She got me started talking to spirits, and that gave me the courage to say in the operating room, to a patient whose heart had stopped, "It's not your time yet. Come on back." His heart started beating again and he survived.

After my folks died, my mystic friend, who does not know my family at all, called me and said, "Your folks are together again and very happy. They are being shown around by a lady who likes chocolate and cigarettes. Do you know who that is?" Before I could respond she said, "It's Elisabeth Kübler-Ross. She's showing your folks around."

So live and learn from your experience and do not let your beliefs close your mind to the truth about life.

DOCTOR'S $\mathcal{R}_x$

Have a meaningful conversation with someone you love. Make it a non-confrontational experience by asking this person two questions: "What animal do you most admire?" and "What attributes does the animal have that capture your admiration?" Listen to his answers, and you can even write them down. When your loved one finishes, explain that the animal is not the significant factor, but that the attributes he described are, because these are this person's own best attributes. Following this revelation, observe where the conversation goes.

You can also ask your loved one what animal he would most like to have in his house. Ask the same question about which of this animal's attributes capture his admiration. When the person is finished answering, explain that he has described his perfect mate or partner.

When I was trying to help one of my patients develop self-esteem, I tried these questions on her. When she answered, "I hate pets and killed my canary," I knew I had my work cut out for me.

Chapter 13

SPIRITUALITY:
FEED YOUR INVISIBLE SELF

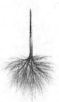

The complete human is one who has faced self-destruction
standing at what William James called 'the perilous edge'...
and has dared to turn back and face the universe.

— BERNIE SIEGEL

Several years ago I fell from our roof, hit my head, and developed amnesia. I soon learned a great deal about the benefits of amnesia. It improved my marriage and family life dramatically when I could not remember the things I used to criticize them for, or the things I had felt angry, resentful, or hurt about. When my memory came back, I had a difficult time with my wife and children because then I remembered all their faults. A therapist friend said she could help me and save me from years of therapy. I asked her how. She wrote something on a piece of paper, handed it to me, and said, "Go home and read this, and live what it says." What she handed me was Corinthians 1:13. It describes what love is and teaches that, although you may appear to have everything, without love, you have nothing.

When you are enlightened, you understand the power of love. Ask yourself, why do we say: kill with kindness, torment with tenderness, love is blind, love thine enemies, and love thy neighbor as thyself? Therein lies the answer to life and enlightenment.

Several years ago there was a series of conferences titled Body and Soul. I always thought people were more likely to bare their souls than their bodies, and so I did one presentation exposing parts of my body to make people aware of how they felt about their own bodies. I felt sad when people came up afterward and told me they were embarrassed or felt bad about their own bodies. To me they seemed perfect. Today, however, I feel much more strongly about getting in touch with and exposing our souls.

We need to respond to our souls and live a soulful life. I can't put into words how I would define *soul*, but it contains our spirit and our deepest needs and meanings related to our life and how we live it. Many of us never speak about these needs and feelings until a crisis or disaster occurs to awaken us to life. I think we know when we are living a soulful life by how our body and our heart feel in relationship to what we are doing, thinking, and feeling. Joseph Campbell said, "If you can see your path laid out in front of you step by step, you know it's not your path. Your own path you make with every step you take. That's why it's your path."[1] He was talking about living a soul-expanding life.

I recently received a book about the benefits of massage from a therapist who was treating someone with what is commonly called multiple personality disorder. Jung suggested — and I am convinced he was right — that we are all multiple personalities. He believed that the goal of each individual is to form a relationship with each of his or her personalities, rather than to suppress one in favor of the other(s). He also believed that in psychoanalysis "the doctor has to establish a relationship with *both* halves of his patient's personality, because only from them both, and not merely from one half with the suppression of the other, can he put together a whole and complete man. The latter alternative is what the patient has been doing all along."[2]

I know — and so does my wife, from the way I behave — that I will do things and speak of things that are beyond my own understanding, and I cannot explain where they came from. I fully accept that within me reside many individuals. When I read this massage therapist's book, I wondered: when you get a massage, do you really know *who* is being massaged, or which of the multiples needs the massage but doesn't get it because a more aggressive personality wants it and takes over the body?

I am not kidding when I say these things. I know from experience and from recorded cases of people with a dissociative disorder that a person can have allergies, diabetes, asthma, and other afflictions associated only with one personality, and a shift to another personality eliminates the disease or problem. But when you think about the roles and situations we become so attached to, perhaps all of us do this to some extent in our lives. We all need to pay attention to the personalities living within us and harmonize them with our soul's desires and needs.

From my perspective, achieving that true balance and using our bodies and light to become soulful in our actions is what life is all about. Think of yourself as a candle. The flame reaches up to the heavens, hoping to reunite with the divine, while the wax and wick represent our earthly bodies and keep us connected and grounded. The flame consumes the wax fuel, and the quality of that fuel is reflected in the purity of the flame. The candle illuminates the world we choose to participate in by sharing our light and love. When we die, that light and love are handed on to future generations. Therein lies our immortality. The light from the candle becomes the pathway to learning about life, just as words are pathways to sharing and understanding ideas.

I create new words on a regular basis, mostly by means of accidents on my computer keyboard. But as Jung said, there are no accidents, so let me share with you the meanings I have found in some of these new words.

When I wrote an article for massage therapists and misspelled *massage*, I created the word *meassage*. It said to me that there is a message in our touch. In other words, every massage given carries a precious message. Recently I was rereading *The Meaning of Love*, edited by Ashley Montagu in 1953, and once again I was impressed by the power of touch to communicate love. Montagu reports that the absence of touch led to an almost 100 percent early mortality rate in children from orphanages where caregivers were fearful that their touch would spread infections from infant to infant and so had avoided touching the babies. Another of my accidental words was GGOD, and to me it describes doing things the way our creator would want us to. What is important is not to know God but to imitate God, and when you do GGod things, you are doing just that.

Then there was *liove*. For me, that unites *living* and *loving*. Those two things should never be separated, but humankind has a problem with this owing to our misunderstanding of separateness. We are not separate, but different parts of one whole. Separation is merely a perception, not a reality. Yin could not exist without yang; the yin/yang symbol shows two shapes with identical outlines that, when inverted and combined, create the circle of wholeness. It is the existence of one that reveals the other. Without one of the two, wholeness no longer exists. So it is with living and loving. Remember, life is not about trying to be perfect but about being complete. Learning this is the soul's work, and when you become aware that nothing is separate, you will be complete; your life will be about living and loving.

I try to learn from many different religions so that I get the message and act as God would want me to act. I was reading something the other day that fit very well with Joseph Campbell's statement that religion may be a misinterpretation of mythology. In other words, there is a message for us in religion that is taught through myths and metaphors, but it is often lost when the writings are interpreted only in the literal sense. What I read said that the word *Torah* should not be translated to mean "the bible" or "the law," but should be understood to mean "teachings or instruction."

When I study a religion, I want to learn how to live my life so that it is meaningful, and the messages taught by that religion's observations or practices enhance my life and the lives of others. When we interpret religious texts as the law, words become our Lord, and we get into conflict with each other over meanings of the words, or who is obeying the law, and how to interpret the law. But when we see religion as something that can guide us, we can have a dialogue about what we see within it and not fight over who is right and who is going to hell.

Finding common themes of guidance in religions, philosophies, or things people write confirms for me that these themes must be meaningful and effective. When I read Joseph Campbell's *The Power of Myth*, I recognized the rebirthing, or born-again, context for survival behavior in his words. He said that heroism is the will to be oneself; the hero is the seeker and the "ism" is the mystery that the seeker seeks to know. In other words, you want to bring forth your true self; you want to be reborn and experience the cycles of change. When you do this, your inner nature is talking. Your soul self — your true self — and its power come forth. This may sound impractical or strictly philosophical, but it is really very basic.

We create our lives by what we decide, think, and act upon each day. We are creating the script for the myth that becomes our life. In my life I have followed what felt right for me, and I am very happy that I did so, instead of worrying about what looked best and appropriate to others. I don't feel as if I have wasted my time here. When I am being interviewed on the radio, somebody always gives me a cue toward the end of the program, saying: "We are running out of time." This motivates me to share that we will all run out of time someday.

Developing your spiritual self is about living; it's about the things you choose to do and fill your mind and body with. But it is also about being — not thinking or doing — just *being*. This brings to mind the story of an old farmer in Somerset, England, who used to sit on a tree stump every evening and gaze across the fields. One day a boy from the village walked by and stopped to ask the old man what he was staring at for so long. The farmer looked at the boy for a long moment. Then with his slow, West Country accent, he said, "Zumm times I sits and thinks, and then zumm times I juz' sits."

We are human beings, not human doings. So don't identify yourself by a role you fulfill; be aware that your divinity defines who you are. Daydreaming and gazing without thought, especially when looking at natural scenes and landscapes, is another way to fulfill your spirit. How many times have you walked past a flowering bush that is humming with bees and other insects while they gather nectar and pollen? Next time, stop for awhile. Just watch and listen. Don't identify the shrub or judge the load each bee carries on its legs; give way to the moment, observe, and forget that you exist. Become nothing and allow everything around you to just be what it is.

When you have a problem, present it to nature and ask for an answer. One time I asked how I could still help people when I was tired of traveling around the world. The answer I received was to spread my seeds as a flower does. I realized then that I didn't have to travel. My words became the seeds, and they didn't need to be delivered in person. My books, CDs, website, and radio and television interviews all became the garden where people could go for help. Another time, when I had a problem that seemed overwhelming, I was shown a skunk cabbage that grew through the pavement and blossomed in the sunlight. I couldn't believe a plant sprout could be strong and wise enough to keep pushing until the pavement cracked.

Our senses of sight, hearing, smell, and touch were designed to feed our bodies with information that helps us survive. When we allow them to bask in beauty and rest in nature, our senses also feed our souls. They transport us, letting us know our connection with life. When we rest our thinking minds and allow nature, the collective consciousness, to stimulate our senses, our thoughts become clear, like the still pond that, undisturbed by wind or current, magnifies the fish swimming below its surface and, at the same time, mirrors the clouds drifting overhead. It is in moments like these that we come to know God.

I have been asked many times to describe what made me aware of my spiritual self and of God, and of the things that changed my perspective. Many of those experiences are shared in this book and in my other writings, such as the time when a voice spoke to me in my state of calm and stillness and told me to go to the shelter where I found the dog Buddy, after writing *Buddy's Candle*; and another time, when my dad appeared to me in a dream after he died and showed me a healthier way to deal with my grief — a way that helped many others heal from theirs; and my experiences with the mystics and psychics who recognized and even drew George, my inner guide, as he stood beside me on the podium.

Perhaps the first time I became aware of my spiritual self was when I was four years old and I was home in bed with one of my frequent ear infections. I took a toy telephone I was playing with and unscrewed the dial. I put all the pieces in my mouth, as I had seen carpenters do with nails so they could hold them there and pull them out one at a time to use. The problem was that I aspirated the pieces and went into laryngospasm. I can still feel my intercostal muscles and diaphragm contracting forcefully, trying to get some air into my lungs, but nothing worked and I was unable to make any sounds to attract help. I had no sense of time, but suddenly realized I was not struggling anymore. I was now at the head of the bed watching myself dying.

I found it fascinating to be free of my body, and it was a blessing. I never stopped to think about how I could still see and think while outside my body. I was feeling sorry that my mother, who was in the kitchen, would find me dead, but I thought it over and found my new state preferable. Intellectually, I chose death over life.

Then the boy on the bed had an agonal seizure, vomited, and all the toy pieces came flying out. He began to breathe again, and I was very angry as I returned to my body against my will. I can still remember yelling, "Who did that?" My thought as a four-year-old was that there was a God who had a schedule, and I wasn't supposed to die now. So an angel apparently did a Heimlich maneuver on me. That's the way I would explain it today.

I really do believe there is a schedule we create unconsciously, and that idea was supported by experiences I had later in life. Twice I have had my car totaled by people driving through red lights and hitting it, and as I said before, I fell off our roof when the top rung on my wooden ladder snapped. In none of these incidents did any significant injury occur to my body.

When considering my life as a child, a husband and father, a healer, an artist, and a writer and speaker, and all the facets of experience that gave me different perspectives, I have come to realize that life is unexplainable. Many of my attitude changes, understandings, and transformations came from the faces and stories of patients and other people who became my teachers. But the knowledge that God is a loving, intelligent, and conscious energy has come to me mostly from dreams, drawings, and past-life and near-death experiences. All of them, I believe, were meant to be my teachers, since I sought none of them and they happened to me in spite of myself.

It doesn't matter if you are reading my books or those of other modern or ancient writers, philosophers, teachers, and guides. None of us have anything new to say about life, love, and matters of the soul; but the way each person expresses this wisdom is different. Each generation tells its own truth, and yet each one repeats ancient wisdom. So read the wisdom of the sages and learn from those who have gone before us. Which path you take makes little difference. Don't wait for a personal disaster to bring you the gift of enlightenment. You may know the saying "If you seek enlightenment, seek it as a man whose hair is on fire seeks water." It takes that kind of desire to truly face the light.

DOCTOR'S R_x

Read, read, and read. Listen to audio books and CDs and read. Study the lives and words of Jesus, Buddha, Muhammad, Epictetus, Lao Tzu, and others. Delve into the poetry and essays of masters such as Dante, Rumi, Gibran, Emerson, and Thoreau. Explore the writings and lectures of modern-day spiritual leaders such as Mother Teresa, the Dalai

Lama, Sri Chinmoy, Joseph Campbell, and Jung. Inspire yourself reading the works of physicists, scientists, and astronauts whose search for
knowledge has broken the illusion of borders between earth and the
rest of the universe and taught us that we are *in* the universe. Enthuse
yourself with delighted expectation. Make reading a daily practice,
even if only for a few minutes each day. Open your mind and read with
a child's curiosity. And reread the same books every few years, because
if they do not become more enlightening, you haven't become more
enlightened.

Epilogue

GRADUATIONS ARE
COMMENCEMENTS

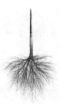

True happiness is to be won by learning to love
with such elevation of spirit as to attain the power to stand up to grief....
Surpass the old love with an even greater new love.

— BENEDETTO CROCE

*A*s the creative effort involved in this book draws to a close, two
things come to mind. Immediately after each of my previous
books went to press, events occurred and stories were shared that I
thought would have been perfect for the book, but it was too late to
include them. *The Art of Healing* will be no different, for when you start
thinking about a certain topic, your consciousness attracts into your life
more of what you think about. It connects with the universal consciousness and changes people's beliefs and experience. It is no coincidence
when that happens, or who it happens to. Jung called it synchronicity.
Another trait my books have in common is summed up by the saying
"It takes a village." I have yet to produce a book all by myself, and I

would be surprised if anyone has ever been able to do so. Just as surgery requires a team of trained, dedicated people, so does a book.

In our final days of editing, events occurred that illustrate and augment the things I have written about in these chapters. This time they happened before we went to press, so I am able to share them with you now.

WALKING THROUGH THE VEIL

Rita was excited to hear that my next book was going to explore creative approaches that delve deeper into the subconscious and that cross boundaries of time, space, and matter. She wrote to me saying that recently she had been finding hearts in nature and photographing them — heart-shaped rocks, a heart-shaped watermelon, and even a three-dimensional heart of meat stuck inside the lid on a can of dog food! Just as my finding pennies reminds me that "in God we trust," for Rita the hearts represent "in love we trust." The most remarkable story she shared with me, however, was about her mother's painting. I'll let Rita tell it in her own words.

My mother was in her late seventies when she took a one-day workshop from a teacher of the Rudolf Steiner method of veil painting. This is a method of watercolor painting that involves using a lot of water and doing layers of color washes down the page. As it dries, you wait to see what emerges. Mom called me after the workshop to say how disappointed she was. All the other students in the class saw trees and many wonderful things emerge from their paintings, but her painting remained just plain color washes, nothing else. She felt she had failed — something she often felt throughout her life.

Mom was an incredible mystic and way ahead of her time spiritually. She had suffered from many tragedies to do with her father and later my dad, but she was a survivor because she always looked ahead and kept going no matter what. She respected all life, all beings, and made no distinctions of any kind. I felt sad for her that after having such hopeful expectations of the veil-painting class, she'd had none of the results the other students achieved.

The next morning she called me in great excitement. "Come and look at my painting," she said. "Come quickly! I can't believe what I'm seeing." I drove there as fast as I possibly could, all the while wondering what in the world could have happened to her painting. When I arrived, I was astonished to see four small human figures emerging from the various layers of color wash. They wore robes and had no faces, and they seemed to be at various depths, with a couple of them farther back and the others moving forward, as if walking toward the front of the painting. My mother swore that the night before, they had not been there. She kept the painting in a safe with her other important papers and documents, and we often pulled it out to look at it together. There was a sense of benevolent energy about the figures that made them seem as if they were really approaching us and weren't just tricks of color and water.

After Mom died, my sister and I had the task of clearing her house. One of the first things I did was go to the safe and look for her veil painting, because I wanted to bring those beautiful beings home with me. As before, it was tucked carefully between her other papers, but when I pulled it out the figures were gone! The painting looked exactly as she had described it after she finished it — plain layers of color wash and nothing else. Along with the four figures, the sense of benevolent energy had left. I realized then that these beings were great spirits; they had come to Mom offering protection and guidance in the next phase of her life's journey. After she passed, their reason for being here was over. Their loving task was completed.

Rita's story did not surprise me. Her mother's benevolent figures might have appeared initially to remind her that she was not a failure and to bestow on her some sense of how beloved she was. But when she died, they became the guides who accompanied her home.

In the beginning of this book I recalled a time that I needed to feel energized and renewed and was out walking the dogs in a local cemetery. I noticed a white object lying on the roadway. I walked over, picked it up, and found that it was a teddy bear with a heart and the words *Love Me* on its chest. I went home renewed. Guides appear in many forms, sometimes in something as simple as a stuffed toy, the words of a song, or a prediction in a horoscope. Sometimes a chain of events is sparked, and the person being guided feels as if she is watching events unfold as another hand makes them happen.

BLUEPRINT THE FUTURE

On December 30, 2012, I forwarded to Cindy, my coauthor on this book, a copy of my numerology reading that had been sent to me. It struck me as being remarkably accurate and contained an exciting New Year's prediction. No coincidence. Because Cindy and I share the same numerology Life Path number, I knew she'd be interested to read what it said:

Numerologists see 2013 as an exciting year when new beginnings are based on an impulse and, like a lineup of tumbling dominoes, are fueled by an energetic chain of events. The person with this Life Path number displays independence and confidence and has a gift for initiating and organizing schemes and working to get things done. This is a time when action must, and will, be taken with extremely positive results. Moving forward, you will create a better life for yourself. Hold on to that which enriches your soul and supports your life goals, but let go of that which is no longer useful or distracts you from your path. Create a new blueprint of what you would like to have happen in your life. This year especially, the dreams that you express in a visual form are the events that you will see unfold.

Cindy has been living and working in the United States for the last ten years. Before that she lived in England, where her daughter, son, and four grandchildren are living now. After reading this numerology report, Cindy confessed that she often feels torn about whether to stay in America or move back to England. Her grandchildren are quickly growing up, and she regrets not being able to participate in their lives. At the same time, she has a deep love for the place where she currently resides; in many ways it feels to her like home. We had just finished working on the edits for the chapter on the drawings, so I said to her, "Draw a picture of yourself in England and another of yourself in the United States."

A few days later, I received an email with only one picture attached (fig. 70). Cindy wrote, "I had no problem drawing the scene of myself in England, but I couldn't begin to imagine what scene to draw here. Looking at this picture makes me feel so happy; I couldn't wait to show it to you. I'm on the left and am supposed to be half running and half squatting so I can hug the kids. But I'm not too good at drawing me squatting on the run. In fact, I'm not sure I can squat on the run! It wasn't until I finished the drawing that I noticed there were no suitcases. I wondered where my bags were, and then I thought, 'Oh good. I'm leaving all that old baggage behind.' And it felt like a new beginning."

After I opened Cindy's scanned drawing, I began writing in a stream-of-consciousness style that lets my intuition communicate at the same time as my analytical mind. My immediate response to her picture was: "Your knees are buckling a little, but you can handle it, and their feet are all turned toward you. Man, this is great. There are eight matching windows on the plane. Every religion has seven days in the week, so the number eight represents a new beginning. There are ten yellow rays on the sun. Ten is a significant number. It comes from the undifferentiated 'no thing' — the zero — and from the 'one' (God), and so, you have creation. (And it is also my birth month!) All your outfits are like a rainbow of healthy colors. Your daughter's husband has bonded with you, with his arm. All the shoes are the same color, as if the family is on the same journey. Everyone has all their senses to communicate with each other. The oldest grandchild is reaching for you, as is your daughter. All your connections with them are right on, with your feet pointed toward each other and the family touching each other. Looks like a great choice."

Doors opened for Cindy when a totally unexpected opportunity for moving back to England presented itself within weeks of her doing this drawing. Her new life will begin in October — the tenth month — and Cindy will be reunited with her family.

When our publishing editor heard this story and saw the drawing, she was delighted. These events couldn't have happened with better timing, nor could there have been a more heartwarming example of how using our creative consciousness helps us to identify our true selves and the future we are creating. They showed how we can set healthy goals and walk into the miracles that bring meaning to our lives. I asked Cindy if her story and drawing could be used in the book. "I guess I'd better call my daughter first and let her know I'm coming," she said, laughing.

As you close the covers of *The Art of Healing*, don't think of it as the end of our time together. Think of it as the beginning of your new journey. You can always visit and read it again. I have learned that if I reread the same books every couple of years, and the books get better each time, it tells me that I am continuing to grow and becoming aware of wisdom that I did not previously notice, owing to my limited state of consciousness at that time.

So, learn from the things I have shared with you. Put them in your pocket or toolbox and continue on your own journey of discovery. Try the various exercises and see what happens. Reparent yourself. Recreate yourself. Find your true path and become who you were always meant to be.

ノotes

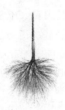

INTRODUCTION. THE BIG QUESTIONS

Epigraph: Plato quoted in M. J. Knight, ed., *A Selection of Passages From Plato for English Readers*, trans. B. Jowett (New York: Macmillan, 1895), vol. 1, p. 2.

1. E. L. Rossi, *The Psychology of Gene Expression* (New York: W. W. Norton, 2002), 4.
2. Ibid., 481.
3. C. Sylvia and W. Novak, *A Change of Heart: A Memoir* (Boston: Little, Brown, 1997), 89.
4. L. McTaggart, *The Field: The Quest for the Secret Force of the Universe*, updated ed. (London: HarperCollins, 2008), 11, the emphasis is mine.
5. W. Bengston and S. Fraser, *The Energy Cure: Unraveling the Mystery of Hands-On Healing* (Louisville, CO: Sounds True, 2010).

CHAPTER 1. THE DOCTOR'S AWAKENING

Epigraph: Rabbi Noah Weinberg, "Way #34: Use Your Inner Guide," Aish.com, January 12, 2000, http://www.aish.com/sp/48w/48950651.html, accessed May 9, 2013.

1. O. C. Simonton, S. Matthews-Simonton, and J. Creighton, *Getting Well*

Again: A Step-by-Step, Self-Help Guide to Overcoming Cancer for Patients and Their Families (New York: Bantam, 1980).

2. C. G. Jung and A. Jaffe, *Memories, Dreams, Reflections* (New York: Random House, 1963).

3. G. M. Furth, *The Secret World of Drawings: A Jungian Approach to Healing through Art* (Boston: Sigo Press, 1988).

4. S. Bach, *Life Paints Its Own Span: On the Significance of Spontaneous Pictures by Severely Ill Children* (Einsiedeln, Switzerland: Daimon Verlag, 1990).

CHAPTER 2. SOURCE, SIGNIFICANCE, AND VALIDITY OF SYMBOLS

Epigraph: Meister Eckhart quoted in *Archive for Research in Archetypal Symbolism*, ed., Ami Ronnberg and Kathleen Martin, *The Book of Symbols: Reflections on Archetypal Images* (Köln: Taschen America, 2010), 6.

1. G. M. Furth, *The Secret World of Drawings: A Jungian Approach to Healing through Art* (Boston: Sigo Press, 1988), 10.

2. C. G. Jung, *The Collected Works of C. G. Jung* (Princeton, NJ: Princeton University Press, 1969), vol. 11, pp. 348–73.

3. J. Campbell and P. Cousineau, *The Hero's Journey: Joseph Campbell on His Life and Work* (Novato, CA: New World Library, 1990); and J. Campbell and B. Moyers, *The Power of Myth* (New York: Anchor, 1991).

4. C. F. Baynes, *The I Ching, or Book of Changes*, trans. R. Wilhelm and C. F. Baynes (Princeton, NJ: Princeton University Press, 1968), xxi–xxv.

5. J. Bartlett, *Familiar Quotations*, 6th ed. (Boston: Little, Brown, 1980), 513.

CHAPTER 3. THE POWER OF VISUALIZATION

Epigraph: Albert Schweitzer quoted in M. Harner, *The Way of the Shaman* (New York: Harper and Row, 1990), 135.

1. A. Pascual-Leone and F. Torres, "Plasticity of the Sensorimotor Cortex Representation of the Reading Finger in Braille Readers," *Brain* 116 (February 1993): 39–52.

Section epigraph: J. Hillman, *Healing Fiction* (Woodstock, CT: Spring Publications, 1983), 47.

CHAPTER 4. DREAMS: THE BRAIN'S CREATIVE WORKSHOP

Epigraph: C. G. Jung, *Jung on Synchronicity and the Paranormal* (London: Routledge, 1997), 73.

1. A. R. Morrison, "The Brain on Night Shift," *Cerebrum* (July 1, 2003), Dana

Foundation website, www.dana.org/news/cerebrum/detail.aspx?id=2950, accessed September 20, 2012.

2. S. Hoffman, "The Message," in *A Book of Miracles: Inspiring True Stories of Healing, Gratitude, and Love*, ed. B. Siegel (Novato, CA: New World Library, 2011), 56–58.

3. C. Sylvia and W. Novak, *A Change of Heart: A Memoir* (Boston: Little, Brown, 1997), 5.

4. G. Holloway, *Dreaming Insights: A 5-Step Plan for Discovering the Meaning in Your Dream* (Portland, OR: Practical Psychology Press, 2002).

CHAPTER 5. DRAWINGS: WHEN CONSCIOUS AND UNCONSCIOUS DISAGREE

Epigraph: T. Guillemets, *The Quote Garden*, www.quotegarden.com/guillemets-quotes.html, accessed September 24, 2012.

1. E. Kübler-Ross, *On Death and Dying* (New York: Scribner, 1997).

2. A. Miller, *Thou Shalt Not Be Aware: Society's Betrayal of the Child* (New York: Farrar, Straus and Giroux, 1998), 315.

3. A. Miller, *Breaking Down the Wall of Silence: The Liberating Experience of Facing Painful Truth* (New York: Penguin, 1996), 153.

4. C. Thomas, "Studies on the Psychological Characteristics of Medical Students" (research paper, Johns Hopkins University School of Medicine, 1964).

5. S. Bach, *Life Paints Its Own Span: On the Significance of Spontaneous Pictures by Severely Ill Children* (Einsiedeln, Switzerland: Daimon Verlag, 1990), 39.

6. C. Dunne, *Carl Jung: Wounded Healer of the Soul* (New York: Parabola Books, 2000), 166.

7. G. M. Furth, *The Secret World of Drawings: A Jungian Approach to Healing through Art* (Boston: Sigo Press, 1988).

CHAPTER 6. INTERPRETING THE DRAWINGS

Epigraph: From Georgia O'Keeffe's statement in the exhibit brochure *Alfred Stieglitz Presents*, quoted in Anna C. Chave, "O'Keeffe and the Masculine Gaze," in *Reading American Art*, ed. M. Doezema and E. Milroy (New Haven, CT: Yale University Press, 1998), 352.

CHAPTER 7. ANIMALS, PSYCHICS, AND INTUITIVES

Epigraph: G. Wendroff, *Heavenletters: Love Letters from God* (Fairfield, IA: 1st World Library, 2004), 144.

1. M. R. Anderson, "The Child Whisperer," in *A Book of Miracles: Inspiring*

True Stories of Healing, Gratitude, and Love, ed. B. Siegel (Novato, CA: New World Library, 2011), 35–38.

2. F. Anderson, excerpt from an unpublished poem, "What If I Were My Cat?" Frances signed her poem "Frances (Feline-Lover) Anderson."

3. G. Corell, *Equestrian Crossings*, 2012, video, Equestrian Crossings website, www.equestriancrossings.com/video/video.html, accessed September 27, 2012.

4. Ibid.

5. T. Crisp, with C. J. Hurn, *No Buddy Left Behind: Bringing U.S. Troops' Dogs and Cats Safely Home from the Combat Zone* (Guilford, CT: Lyons Press, 2012), dust jacket.

6. Ibid., 136, 244. The quotes are taken from a taped interview by Cynthia Hurn, December 3, 2010.

7. B. Siegel and M. G. Stein, *Buddy's Candle* (Victoria, BC: Trafford, 2008).

8. A. Kinkade, *The Language of Miracles: A Celebrated Psychic Teaches You to Talk to Animals* (Novato, CA: New World Library, 2006).

9. Olga's story is told in E. Cerutti, *Olga Worrall: Mystic with the Healing Hands* (New York: Harper and Row, 1975).

CHAPTER 8. LAUGH OUT LOUD

Epigraph: B. Siegel, *Prescriptions for Living: Inspirational Lessons* (New York: HarperCollins, 1998), 15.

1. Norman's story is told in N. Cousins, *Anatomy of an Illness as Perceived by the Patient* (New York: W. W. Norton, 2005).

2. D. Spoto, *Notorious: The Life of Ingrid Bergman* (Cambridge: DaCapo Press, 2001), 165, the emphasis is mine.

3. B. Siegel, "Divorce," in *Prescription for Living: Inspirational Lessons for a Joyful, Loving Life* (New York: HarperCollins, 1999), 16.

CHAPTER 9. FAKE IT TILL YOU MAKE IT

Epigraph: Helen Keller quoted in W. Fogg, *One Thousand Sayings of History: Presented as Pictures in Prose* (Boston: Beacon Press, 1929), 17.

1. Child Welfare Information Gateway, *Understanding the Effects of Maltreatment on Brain Development* (Washington, DC: Department of Health and Human Services, 2009), www.childwelfare.gov/pubs/issue_briefs/brain_development/brain_development.pdf, accessed September 24, 2012. And for further information and resources on this subject, see the U.S. Department of Health and Human Services website: www.childwelfare.gov/pubs/can_info_packet.pdf.

2. Membership statistics retrieved from Alcoholics Anonymous, www.aa.org /en_pdfs/smf-53_en.pdf, accessed February 12, 2013.
3. T. Hunter, "Rock Me to Sleep," from *Bits & Pieces*, 1977, CD, www.tomhunter.com/store/bits&pieces.htm, accessed September 24, 2012.

CHAPTER 10. WORDS CAN KILL OR CURE

Epigraph: J. Hillman, *Healing Fiction* (Woodstock, CT: Spring Publications, 1983), 46.
1. Lao Tzu, *Tao Te Ching*, trans. S. Mitchell (New York: HarperCollins, 2000), 44.

CHAPTER 11. CHOOSE LIFE

Epigraph: Bernie Siegel
1. B. Klopfer, "Psychological Variables in Human Cancer," *Journal of Projective Techniques* 21, no. 4 (December 1957): 331–40.

CHAPTER 12. END-OF-LIFE TRANSITIONS

Epigraph: K. Gibran, *The Prophet* (Ware, Hertfordshire: Wordsworth Editions, 1997), 50.
1. Quoted in F. Hesselbein, "A Splendid Torch," *Leader to Leader* 22 (Fall 2001): 4–5.
2. T. Hunter, "Rock Me to Sleep," from *Bits & Pieces*, 1977, CD, www.tomhunter.com/store/bits&pieces.htm, accessed September 24, 2012.

CHAPTER 13. SPIRITUALITY: FEED YOUR INVISIBLE SELF

Epigraph: Bernie Siegel
1. J. Campbell, *Reflections on the Art of Living: A Joseph Campbell Companion*, ed. D. K. Osbon (New York: HarperCollins, 1991), 22.
2. C. G. Jung, *The Undiscovered Self*, trans. R. F. C. Hull (London: Penguin, 1958), 87.

EPILOGUE. GRADUATIONS ARE COMMENCEMENTS

Epigraph: Benedetto Croce quoted in L. Chang, *Wisdom for the Soul* (Washington, DC: Gnosophia, 2006), 484.

Index

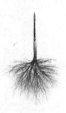

About Bernie S. Siegel, MD

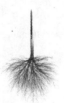

*B*ernie S. Siegel, MD, is a well-known proponent of integrative and holistic approaches to healing that heal not just the body but also the mind and soul. Bernie, as his friends and patients call him, attended Colgate University and studied medicine at Cornell University Medical College. His surgical training took place at Yale–New Haven Hospital, West Haven Veterans Hospital, and the Children's Hospital of Pittsburgh. In 1978 Bernie pioneered a new approach to group and individual cancer therapy called Exceptional Cancer Patients (ECaP), which utilized patients' drawings, dreams, and feelings, and he broke new ground in facilitating important patient lifestyle changes and engaging the patient in the healing process.

Bernie retired from his general and pediatric surgical practice in 1989. Always a strong advocate for his patients, he has since dedicated himself to humanizing the medical establishment's approach to patients and empowering patients to play a vital role in the process of self-induced healing to achieve their greatest potential. He continues to run support groups and is an active speaker, traveling around the world to address patient and caregiver groups. As the author of several books — including *Love, Medicine & Miracles*; *Peace, Love & Healing*; *How to Live between Office Visits*; *365 Prescriptions for the Soul*; *Faith, Hope & Healing*; and *A Book of Miracles* — Bernie has been at the forefront of spiritual and medical ethics issues of our day. He has been named one of the top twenty Spiritually Influential Living People by *Watkins' Mind Body Spirit* magazine (London). Bernie and his wife (and occasional coauthor), Bobbie, live in a suburb of New Haven, Connecticut. They have five children, eight grandchildren, four cats, two dogs, and much love. Visit his website at www.berniesiegelmd.com.

About Cynthia J. Hurn

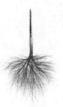

Freelance writer and editor Cynthia J. Hurn is a coauthor of the nonfiction book *No Buddy Left Behind: Bringing U.S. Troops' Dogs and Cats Safely Home from the Combat Zone*. Her studies in psychology, counseling, and creative writing, plus her work with animals and rescued wild birds, bring a unique mixture of science, heart, and soul to her writing.

NEW WORLD LIBRARY is dedicated to publishing books and other media that inspire and challenge us to improve the quality of our lives and the world.

We are a socially and environmentally aware company, and we strive to embody the ideals presented in our publications. We recognize that we have an ethical responsibility to our customers, our staff members, and our planet.

We serve our customers by creating the finest publications possible on personal growth, creativity, spirituality, wellness, and other areas of emerging importance. We serve New World Library employees with generous benefits, significant profit sharing, and constant encouragement to pursue their most expansive dreams.

As a member of the Green Press Initiative, we print an increasing number of books with soy-based ink on 100 percent postconsumer-waste recycled paper. Also, we power our offices with solar energy and contribute to nonprofit organizations working to make the world a better place for us all.

Our products are available
in bookstores everywhere.
For our catalog, please contact:

New World Library
14 Pamaron Way
Novato, California 94949

Phone: 415-884-2100 or 800-972-6657
Catalog requests: Ext. 50
Orders: Ext. 52
Fax: 415-884-2199
Email: escort@newworldlibrary.com

To subscribe to our electronic newsletter, visit:
www.newworldlibrary.com

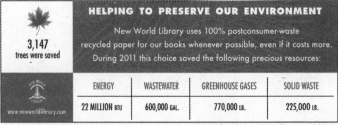

HELPING TO PRESERVE OUR ENVIRONMENT

3,147 trees were saved

New World Library uses 100% postconsumer-waste recycled paper for our books whenever possible, even if it costs more. During 2011 this choice saved the following precious resources:

	ENERGY	WASTEWATER	GREENHOUSE GASES	SOLID WASTE
www.newworldlibrary.com	22 MILLION BTU	600,000 GAL.	770,000 LB.	225,000 LB.

Environmental impact estimates were made using the Environmental Defense Fund Paper Calculator @ www.papercalculator.org.